NEW TRICKS

ABOUT THE AUTHOR

Emeritus Professor Richard G. Larkins, AO

Richard Graeme Larkins was born in Melbourne in 1943. He graduated as the top medical graduate at the University of Melbourne in 1966. He was awarded a PhD by the University of London in 1974. His career since then has encompassed clinical medicine, specialising in diabetes and endocrinology, clinical and laboratory research, medical education at undergraduate and postgraduate levels, medical and university leadership. He has held many senior academic and leadership roles including James Stewart Professor of Medicine at the University of Melbourne, dean of the Faculty of Medicine, Dentistry and Health Sciences at the University of Melbourne and vice-chancellor and president of Monash University. In addition, he has been chair of the National Health and Medical Research Council, president of the Royal Australasian College of Physicians, chair of Universities Australia and chair of both the Medical School and Specialist Education Accreditation Committee of the Australian Medical Council. He has been a member of the National Aboriginal and Torres Strait Islander Health Council and on two occasions a member of the Prime Minister's Science, Engineering and Innovation Council. He has held numerous other posts on government committees in Australia and Asia.

He has published 200 refereed research papers, reviews and chapters and has co-authored or edited five books. He is a fellow of the Royal Australasian College of Physicians, the Royal College of Physicians, the Royal College of Physicians of Ireland, the Academies of Medicine of Singapore and of Malaysia and of the Academy of Technological Sciences and Engineering. He is an honorary fellow of the American College of Physicians, the Ceylon College of Physicians and the Royal College of Physicians of Thailand. He has been awarded honorary Doctor of Laws degrees at both Monash University and the University of Melbourne. He has been awarded the Eric Susman Prize for Medical Research by the Royal Australasian College of Physicians, the Sir William Upjohn Medal for Distinguished Service to Medicine and the Brownless Medal for outstanding contribution to the Melbourne Medical School and a Centenary of Federation Medal. He is a fellow of Melbourne's Trinity College, an officer in the general division of the Order of Australia and an emeritus professor at Monash University. He remains active in a number of leadership roles in health and education.

NEW TRICKS

REFLECTIONS ON A LIFE IN MEDICINE AND TERTIARY EDUCATION

RICHARD LARKINS

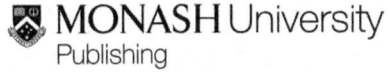

© Copyright 2015 Richard Larkins

All rights reserved. Apart from any uses permitted by Australia's Copyright Act 1968, no part of this book may be reproduced by any process without prior written permission from the copyright owners. Inquiries should be directed to the publisher.

Monash University Publishing
Matheson Library and Information Services Building
40 Exhibition Walk
Monash University
Clayton, Victoria 3800, Australia
www.publishing.monash.edu

Every effort has been made to trace owners of copyright material, but in some cases this has not proved possible. The publishers would be interested to hear from any copyright holders not here acknowledged.

Monash University Publishing brings to the world publications which advance the best traditions of humane and enlightened thought.

www.publishing.monash.edu/books/nt-9781922235435.html

Series: Biography

Design: Les Thomas

Front cover image: Portrait of Richard Larkins by Juan Ford. Reproduced with permission.

National Library of Australia Cataloguing-in-Publication entry:
Author: Larkins, Richard, author.
Title: New tricks : reflections on a life in medicine and tertiary education / Richard Larkins.
ISBN: 9781922235435 (paperback).
Subjects: Larkins, Richard.
Universities and colleges--Faculty--Australia.
Academic achievement--Philosophy.
Educational leadership--Philosophy.
Medical policy--Australia.
Medicine--Research--Australia.
Conduct of life.
Dewey Number: 378.12

Printed in Australia by Griffin Press an Accredited ISO AS/NZS 14001:2004 Environmental Management System printer.

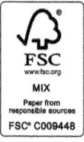

The paper this book is printed on is certified against the Forest Stewardship Council ® Standards. Griffin Press holds FSC chain of custody certification SGS-COC-005088. FSC promotes environmentally responsible, socially beneficial and economically viable management of the world's forests.

CONTENTS

About the author ii

Preface vii

1. Context 1
2. Undergraduate at the University of Melbourne 6
3. Internship and clinical training at the Royal Melbourne Hospital ... 14
4. London 21
5. The senior medical staff of the Royal Melbourne Hospital 31
6. The Repatriation General Hospital Heidelberg 36
7. Saudi Arabia, 1981 41
8. The James Stewart Chair of Medicine, University of Melbourne, at the Royal Melbourne Hospital 45
9. China, 1985 51
10. Casemix funding and the 'crisis' in the hospitals in the 1990s 58
11. Medical education, the medical workforce and the Doherty Committee of Inquiry 68
12. The Medical School Accreditation Committee of the Australian Medical Council 75
13. Deputy Dean of the Faculty of Medicine, Dentistry and Health Sciences at the University of Melbourne, and reform of the medical curriculum 81
14. Dean of the Faculty of Medicine, Dentistry and Health Sciences at the University of Melbourne 93
15. Chair of the National Health and Medical Research Council 114

16. The National Aboriginal and Torres Strait Islander Health Council and Indigenous Health 125

17. President of the Royal Australasian College of Physicians 129

18. Appointment at Monash University 139

19. Early days at Monash University. 148

20. The end of the honeymoon – student riots and a flashback to the 1960s 156

21. Administration and finance. 161

22. Research and scholarship 171

23. Education 179

24. The Victorian campuses of Monash University. 185

25. Monash University Malaysia, Sunway Campus 198

26. Monash South Africa 203

27. Monash University in Europe. 209

28. IITB-Monash Research Academy, India 214

29. Monash University in China. 221

30. Other international activities of Monash University. 227

31. Universities Australia 236

32. Farewell to Monash. 246

33. Life after Monash 249

34. Final Reflections 255

Index 257

PREFACE

'High above the hushed crowd, Rex tried to remain focused. Still, he couldn't shake one nagging thought: he was an old dog and this was a new trick.'

These words lay beneath a Gary Larson cartoon showing a dog riding a unicycle on a tightrope in a circus big top while juggling balls with its front paws, swinging a hoop round its middle, balancing a jug on its head and holding a cat in its mouth. The card with the cartoon was sent to me by my long-time scientific colleague, Marjorie Dunlop, to mark my transition from dean of the Faculty of Medicine, Dentistry and Health Sciences at the University of Melbourne to vice-chancellor and president of Monash University in 2003. I had just turned sixty and this was indeed a new trick.

I started writing these reflections three days after I completed my term at Monash University. I was entering the next phase of my life. It would be studded with a variety of interesting and challenging part-time activities. I thought it an appropriate time to reflect on the tricks I have learnt both as a young dog and an old dog and the experiences I have had in an adult lifetime spent in medicine, research, health policy and higher education.

My aim is to provide a personal account rather than a detailed historical document. I will intersperse my account of how things have transpired with a critique of how our systems work and could be improved. I will try to be as frank and open as I can while respecting confidentiality and individual feelings.

I acknowledge the role that so many have played in what has been for me an incredibly rewarding and fulfilling career and life. This includes my medical and research mentors and colleagues, the PhD and other research students I have supervised, the medical students and graduates I have taught and my academic and administrative colleagues at the University of Melbourne and Monash University. My executive assistants, Liz Mobilio at the University of Melbourne and Kerrie Edwards at Monash were highly efficient, hardworking and supportive.

Most of all I have been extremely fortunate to have had an extremely supportive family.

NEW TRICKS

My mother Peg Lusink was inspirational in the way she regrouped, retrained and carved out a spectacular career for herself after the early death of my father and did this while caring for three teenage sons.

My wife Caroline and our three daughters, Sarah, Fiona and Kate and now their husbands and children have been a constant source of happiness and comfort. Caroline has provided the love and stability necessary to compensate for the distractions from a career too full. She deserves as much credit as me for anything I have been fortunate to achieve.

Chapter 1

CONTEXT

'They said we were mad to get married when we did, but we had nineteen wonderful years together that we would not have had.'

Those words, spoken by my mother and overheard from the top of the stairs of our house, told me that my father, Graeme, had died. It was 1959. He was thirty-seven, a chain smoker and severely hypertensive, and he had had a massive subarachnoid haemorrhage (burst aneurysm) that morning. I was sixteen, my two brothers John and Stephen, eighteen and thirteen.

My father was a quiet, big man who had met my mother Peg at a cadet dance at Melbourne Grammar School. They married shortly after they started university when they were both eighteen. My mother abandoned her law course and worked as a nurse to support her new family and dedicated the first phase of her life to her husband and children.

Graeme's death transformed our family's life and probably had more of an influence on my own life than I cared to admit at the time.

My father came from a broken family, the only son of Bill, a lovable but roguish insurance salesman and Chlothilde. Chlothilde came from a family involved in a successful stone masonry business and she established a prominent toy shop, Tim the Toyman, in Melbourne. Graeme was educated at Melbourne Grammar School, was academically gifted and rowed in the winning 1938 Head of the River crew. He went to Melbourne University to study medicine at sixteen and, despite the distractions of marriage and children, finished in the top two or three of his year.

My mother's father, Edward Rosanove, was born in Palestine, as his Jewish parents fled from one of the pogroms in the Ukraine. His family moved to Australia when he was an infant, initially to Broken Hill and later Adelaide. He studied medicine at the University of Melbourne and became a successful dermatologist.

My mother's mother, Joan Rosanove, came from Ballarat, one of nine children in a secular Jewish family. Her father, Mark Lazarus, was a respected solicitor. Although never appearing to her grandchildren to be a driven woman, she must have been, as she commuted daily by train to Melbourne to study law through the articled clerk pathway. She later became the first female barrister in Victoria and the first woman Queen's Counsel in the state. She was a pioneer for female lawyers and became a celebrated barrister specialising in matrimonial law. A building housing legal chambers has been named in her honour (Joan Rosanove Chambers).

After completion of his compressed war-time medical course, my father enlisted in the navy. While waiting to be assigned, he took up a six month locum position in Walwa on the upper Murray river. The war then ended and as the doctor in nearby Corryong was leaving, he bought the practice and was the sole doctor in the region for the next eight years. Corryong is an idyllic town at the foothills of the Snowy Mountains, virtually drought-proof and surrounded by fertile grazing land.

Despite the challenges and satisfaction that come from rural general practice, Graeme wished to pursue further medical study and to become a consultant physician. We moved to Melbourne in 1952, and my father flew first to the USA and then to the United Kingdom to undertake specialist training as a physician. After about three months away, he telegrammed to say that he was lonely. My mother, in a typically impulsive and wonderfully irrational decision, decided that we should all join him in London. Impossibly, she made all the arrangements for us to sail to London, packed us up, and we sailed for London on the *Strathaird* twenty-four hours after she had decided we would go.

The three boys were enrolled at St David's School in Queensgate. For three young Australians used to the freedom of life in the country, St David's was very repressive. It was run by a family, the Durnfords, and would not have been out of place in one of Dickens' novels. Still, the strict discipline ensured sound education and a flying start in French and Latin, which were not to appear in the Australian curriculum till years later.

Despite his period away from study and the lack of clinical experience in a teaching hospital environment, Graeme eventually passed the tough examinations to become a member of both the London and Edinburgh

CHAPTER 1

colleges of physicians. When he returned to Australia, he added the membership of the Royal Australasian College of Physicians.

During his time in the USA and in the UK, he had been particularly impressed by the emerging specialty of geriatric medicine and decided to bring some of the new approaches to the care of the sick elderly to Australia. The emphasis on rehabilitation following stroke and on the role of diet and exercise in preserving health and preventing disease in the elderly became particular interests.

Graeme was the first consultant physician in Victoria to identify himself as a geriatrician. He introduced active rehabilitation to Mount Royal Hospital for the Aged and was responsible for the design of the rehabilitation building. He declined its directorship, as he wished to continue in part-time private practice. A wing of Mount Royal is now named after him.

My father had a particular affinity with the elderly and I remember accompanying him on Christmas morning ward rounds at Mount Royal, where the adoration of his patients was moving. He continued to work half-time in private practice and as an outpatient physician at the Alfred.

Shortly before his sudden death, I recall him saying, 'I should not be paid for what I am doing – I enjoy it so much.' I suspect that this comment subliminally led me to make the decision to study medicine, and perhaps that decision was strengthened by Graeme's death.

Following my father's death, my mother worked part-time and recommenced her law studies. She graduated in five years and also met another mature age law student, Theo Lusink, whom she was to marry, and they have lived happily together for forty-nine years. My mother, Peg Lusink, after a period as a solicitor and as a barrister, was appointed as one of the foundation justices of the Family Court, a position she filled with distinction for many years before retiring. She then had three years as a professor of law at Bond University, specialising in mediation. Peg is irrepressibly enthusiastic and extroverted, immensely loyal to her family and always working on new projects. She remains active in retirement, having recently moved back to Melbourne from Benalla.

I finished my schooling at Melbourne Grammar in the year following my father's death, coming joint dux of the school, winning the BHP Prize for top in the state for the aggregate matriculation marks for physics, chemistry and a branch of maths and winning the exhibition for top in the state for physics as well as a general exhibition. I loved sport, rowed in the second eight and played football in the fourth eighteen – undistinguished but wildly enthusiastic.

I do remember with pride two of my early rebellions against the establishment. The first was my wish to resign from the cadets because I did not believe in war. I was shamed by my housemaster into staying on, but chose to go into the non-combatant field security area. I gained my revenge by losing a whole platoon because of my total lack of a sense of direction.

The second episode was also trivial. We were told that we all had to buy Flanders poppies to commemorate November 11 and the servicemen who had given their lives for Australia. I said to the master involved that this was wrong. We should want to buy the poppies, but to make it compulsory totally defeated the purpose. If we had to do it, it meant nothing. It was a subtle point in the conformist atmosphere of private schools for boys in the 1950s.

At that time, it was usual for boys to do two years' matriculation to 'broaden them, give leadership experience and to allow them to achieve their potential at sport'. Our somewhat straitened circumstances, which had seen us sell our newly completed house in Toorak and move to more modest (although hardly deprived) quarters in South Yarra, prevented me from having that experience, so I started at the University of Melbourne in 1961 – coincidentally the year that the new university, Monash, took its first students.

I left school with sage words of advice from the imposing headmaster of Melbourne Grammar School. Brian Hone was a much admired and inspirational headmaster and I know that I and my fellow students learnt much from him. It is ironic that there are only three bits of specific advice that I can recall.

The first came in our last assembly: 'Remember, boys, it is an unjust world;' sound and helpful words which have prevented me railing against perceived injustices from that time on.

The next two came when he conducted classes in religious instruction. I am not sure of their relevance to religion and I am afraid I ignored both of them. 'Do not drink spirits until you are thirty', and 'When you are thinking of getting married, look at your prospective bride's mother – that is what she will be like in twenty years' time'.

CHAPTER 1

In the case of the last bit of 'advice', although my mother-in-law, Betty Cust, was a redoubtable and admirable woman who died in 2014 at the age of 97, my wife is very much from the other side of the family gene pool and has not in any way become like her mother.

Chapter 2

UNDERGRADUATE AT THE UNIVERSITY OF MELBOURNE

I was fortunate to win a scholarship to attend Trinity College, a residential college associated with the University of Melbourne, to study medicine. Although Monash University and its medical school had opened that year, I cannot recall giving it serious consideration – the University of Melbourne was so well established, my older brother was there and it had for a century been the logical next step for Melbourne Grammar boys smart enough to get there and without either a Western District property or a seat on the stock exchange to ease them into a life of comfort.

University life in those days was privileged and enjoyable. Tweed sports coats and ties, sherry parties, tennis days with the ladies of Janet Clarke Hall and program dance nights. It was an Antipodean replica of Oxford and Cambridge in a city not yet sufficiently infused with the vigour from our southern European and later Asian immigrants to define a more individual character.

College life, while tending to isolate students from the more general university environment, had the advantage of bringing students from all disciplines together in a stimulating intellectual and social mix. It also provided wonderful opportunities for sporting activities, and even a mediocre sportsperson such as me could represent the college at rowing, football and golf. It provided an environment for smart people to do clever and wicked things. A notable feature of our first year at Trinity was the celebrated 'fixing' of Juttoddie by the bookmakers.

Juttoddie was the traditional handicap race around the college buildings for the freshmen. They were required to run in their academic gowns, carrying a prescribed handicap of a number of bricks around an obstacle course. Betting on the race added to the excitement. Interference with water

CHAPTER 2

bombing and the like was common. In our fresher year, there was a short-priced favourite. The bookmakers stood to lose heavily if he won. So they did what any sensible bookie would do in such circumstances. They hired a helicopter and its pilot and, at just the right moment in the race, landed, abducted the favourite who was leading and flew him away. Dangerous, stupid and childish, but great fun.

Preclinical medical education at that time was, by and large, dreadful. It was very traditional, with the first year consisting of pre-medicine, a recapitulation of physics and chemistry and, for those like me who had not taken it at matriculation, an introduction to biology, including botany. Minimal efforts were made to make the subjects relevant to medicine and if it had not been for the alternative attractions of college life, with its sport and a newly discovered and liberated social life, it would have been very boring.

Second year at least embraced subjects that we could see were relevant to medicine, although they were taught in a way intended to highlight the beauty and aesthetics of the discipline rather than to draw any particular relevance to medical disease or treatment. We learnt by rote the intermediates of the Krebs cycle and other arcane details of biochemistry. We dissected out methodically and often with imagination rather than accuracy the branches of the peripheral nerves and arteries. We learnt the markings on our sets of bones which represented the insertions of muscles and attachments of ligaments.

Our lecturers represented an era where what they said was gospel and how they said it was their business. There were no evaluation of the lecturers by the students and we could not even vote with our feet, as we had assigned alphabetical seating so that our presence at the lectures could be confirmed, and it was compulsory.

I particularly recall three lecturers whose idiosyncrasies typify university education at that time.

One was a histology and embryology lecturer. A very distinguished grey-haired man who was apparently pathologically shy, rumoured to be due to trauma in the war. He would come into the lecture theatre, immediately turn to the board and then in meticulous detail draw the particular histological or embryological dissections using coloured chalk to distinguish the tissues and layers. When he was finished, he would leave, avoiding the necessity of speaking to us.

A second was an anatomy professor. He was more interested in medical history than he was in anatomy at that stage of his career. I particularly remember one lecture. The topic was the clavicle (collarbone). He came into the lecture theatre, held up a clavicle and started to speak at full speed, pointing out the markings of the relevant attachments. These were quite invisible to all the students in the lecture theatre. He proceeded apparently without drawing breath (although he must have done, as he was quite obese). After about fifteen minutes, he turned on his heel and departed, leaving us bemused and knowing no more about the clavicle than we did before the lecture. Of course, we then learnt all the attachments by heart from *Gray's Anatomy* and remembered them just long enough for the examinations.

We also had lectures from the renowned 'Pansy' Wright, a celebrated physiologist. He was an advocate of human rights and had gained considerable publicity and notoriety by steadfastly supporting Sidney Orr, a professor of philosophy at the University of Tasmania, who had been sacked for having an affair with one of his students. As described in Peter McPhee's excellent biography, Pansy was a dishevelled, disorganised man with an acerbic, ribald wit. His lectures were even more disorganised than his appearance and, although they contained occasional pearls, they were mostly unintelligible.

I say this in no way to disparage the individuals I have mentioned, who were all people of considerable achievement. Rather, the point I wish to make is that the quality of medical education at our universities has improved enormously over the last few decades. There have been specific changes in approach to medical education, but over and above this, the general quality of university teaching has improved in all disciplines, with attention paid to developing the skills of lecturers, new educational technology and student feedback to lecturers.

Dissection of the human body was part of the ritual of the preclinical years. A vast amount of time was devoted to this. In retrospect it was totally disproportionate to the value of the process. At the end of second year, the top six students in anatomy were granted the status of prosectors and shared a body to dissect in the following year. One of my fellow prosectors was Geoffrey Edelsten, who was to become the most (in)famous graduate in our year. He was engaging, articulate, intelligent and hardworking, with a hunger for making money. By the time we finished our course, he had started an agency for pop stars. In our first year residency (internship), he had started a locum service, and he later pioneered just about every form of get-

CHAPTER 2

rich scheme for doctors in Australia, including chains of twenty-four-hour clinics, laser tattoo removal, pathology services, including paternity genetic testing and many others. He had many run-ins with the medical boards of two states, was run off the road by a hit man and owned the Sydney Swans, an AFL football team.

The clinical years of the course were conducted in the time-honoured hospital-based student clerkships. The obvious relevance, the direct contact with patients and the confrontation with suffering and death all concentrated our minds to a much greater extent than the preclinical years. Our teachers were, for the most part, the 'honoraries', the consultant physicians and surgeons who spent most of their time in private practice and part of their time in pro bono work in public hospitals. There they were involved in teaching the medical students and supervising the interns, residents and registrars undertaking specialist training as well as providing consultant care to the inpatients and outpatients.

In relatively recent times, this system had been complemented by the creation of clinical academic units in medicine, surgery, paediatrics, obstetrics and gynaecology, psychiatry and radiology. In the case of medicine and surgery at the Royal Melbourne Hospital, the foundation professor of medicine was a young Englishman, Richard Lovell, and the foundation professor of surgery, a delightful Scot, Maurice Ewing. They had taken up their positions in 1956, eight years before we started our clinical years in 1964. Perhaps not surprisingly, these foreign imports were viewed with suspicion and treated with disrespect by some of the firmly embedded honoraries, who were used to being the established authorities. They had tended to use their experience and stated dogma as the basis for their teaching rather than the newfangled approach based on research and evidence. Gradually, the new professors earned respect, but it was a long slow process.

One episode in particular illustrates the difficulty that faced the new professors. Some of the consultants at the Royal Melbourne Hospital had appointments at the Peter MacCallum Cancer Clinic, then located downtown in William Street. Maurice Ewing was one of these and when our fourth-year group of seven students was rostered to his unit, we accompanied him to Peter Mac. Things were quiet in his clinic, so he suggested we spend some time in an adjoining clinic with Sir Benjamin Rank. We duly did, awed to be in the presence of the revered plastic surgeon with a celebrated period of war service and world-renowned for his surgical expertise. We stood quietly watching the great man at work. For twenty minutes he showed no sign of being aware of our presence. Then our hearts leapt as he spoke to us, albeit without looking up.

'You are Professor Ewing's students, aren't you?'

'Yes', we said enthusiastically, thinking that this would be the prelude to his unveiling the secrets of distinguishing benign from malignant skin lesions, which seemed to be his task at the time. We waited for the next words from the great man.

'I am not Professor Ewing.' Humiliated, we slunk off.

I should add that in my years as a resident and young consultant at Royal Melbourne Hospital, I found that Sir Benjamin, although taciturn and gruff, was in fact a generous man and very supportive of education.

The professor of obstetrics and gynaecology was a particularly legendary character. Lance Townsend was a disciplinarian of the old school, believing in regimentation. This was reflected in immaculate white uniforms for the students, strict rules about behaviour in the student residences, ritual humiliation for anyone who may have looked imperfectly shaved and absolute dogmatism in his teaching. He later became dean of the faculty and ruled it with a similar rod of iron. Most of us learnt a lot of obstetrics and gynaecology, albeit largely through fear rather than because of an innate love for the subject or the way it was then taught.

In complete contrast, the professor of paediatrics was a gentle and caring man, Vernon Collins. He impressed us enormously by addressing us with our names from the first morning we were at the Royal Children's Hospital. It was quite a feat to be able to do so from the poor quality 'mug shots' taken when we commenced our course that he must have used to identify us. We all loved paediatrics and the part played as a role model by Vernon Collins was significant in this.

We were privileged to have one or more lectures from individuals who had made significant contributions to medical knowledge and treatment. John Cade had discovered the role of lithium in the treatment of bipolar or manic depressive illness. This was the first truly effective form of drug treatment for psychiatric disease. His presentation of a hypomanic patient at Royal Park Hospital was mesmerising. Kate Campbell had described the role of the administration of 100 per cent oxygen in causing retrolental fibrosis and thus blindness in premature infants and thereby altered practice and prevented further cases of tragic blindness in children. Priscilla Kincaid-Smith, later to

CHAPTER 2

become a respected colleague, described the role of combination analgesics in causing a particular type of renal failure, at that time very common. This led to alterations in formulation of over-the-counter painkillers and the elimination of this prominent cause of renal failure.

At Trinity College we were very fortunate to have two outstanding teachers, both named Ian McKenzie. We had heard from the medical students in the year ahead that Ian McKenzie gave outstanding medical tutorials. We looked up the medical directory and approached Ian (H.) McKenzie. He was a physician at Prince Henry's Hospital, which was a teaching hospital for Monash University. He must have been surprised and perhaps a little flattered to be approached by students from the University of Melbourne, but he gave us clinical tutorials for our final year at Prince Henry's Hospital on Saturdays. They were outstanding and he continued to give tutorials to Trinity medical students for many years. Medical scholarships at Trinity College are now named in his honour. The other Ian (F.C.) McKenzie was eventually also enlisted. He gave us simply superb theoretical tutorials in college. He later became a distinguished immunology and cancer researcher and director of the Austin Research Institute.

University was also notable as the time I met my future wife, Caroline. I had admired her from afar for the three years she had been in Trinity's sister college, Janet Clarke Hall (JCH), studying arts and psychology. Eventually, I plucked up courage and asked her out to dinner. Unbeknownst to me, she had been to the same restaurant with another suitor the night before. I missed the telling wink to her from the waiter. We had a good conversation at dinner and I returned her to JCH with the thought that I could see why she was being pursued by a number of my Trinity colleagues and others, but she was clearly out of my league and would not be interested in me.

On Saturday, two days later, I discovered a blue glove on the floor of the passenger side of my old FJ Holden (this was a long time ago!). As I had driven some of my medical student group to a tutorial the day before, I was not sure whose glove it was and decided to ask them on Monday if it belonged to one of them. On Sunday evening, Caroline knocked on the door of my study to ask me if I had seen her glove. Naturally, I invited her in – and the rest, as they say, is history. Years later, she admitted it was a deliberate ploy to ensure that she had an excuse to come and see me again, perhaps sensing that as it had taken me three years to ask her out once, it may not happen again! I was a pawn in the face of such feminine guile, but I have forever been grateful for Caroline's creativity and initiative (along with her other qualities).

After an appropriate period of courtship, I asked her delightful father, Eric, for her hand and somewhat naively expected to be welcomed into the family. Instead, I was escorted into the study and asked whether I could keep Caroline in the way to which she was accustomed. I looked around and clearly the answer was no. Did I have life insurance? I asked what was there to insure. I was penniless, fatherless and, at that stage, jobless. My ancestry must have seemed, to this conventional Anglo-Protestant household, challenging at best. But to my future father-in-law's credit, having gone through the formalities and despite, I am sure, considerable reservations, he consented. We became engaged as I was starting final year medicine, when I was twenty-two and Caroline twenty-one.

As a condition of their acquiescence, Caroline's parents promptly took her away for the grand overseas tour. She was introduced to a range of more eligible potential husbands, but stood firm in her somewhat irrational choice. My sole comfort in the years of struggle I put Caroline through over the next few decades was that at some moment of insight on my part and blind love on hers, I declared that I was not going to be the sort of doctor that would make a lot of money and she said that it did not matter!

Final year seemed to take an eternity. In those days, continuing assessment was irrelevant. Everything depended on the final examination. There had been no examinations since the clinical years started two and a quarter years before. Finals started with seven three-hour written papers over three and a half days covering the major clinical subjects. It was a test of endurance as much as knowledge. Clinical and oral examinations followed over the next couple of weeks.

Caroline and I were due to be married immediately after the examinations. Unfortunately, I miscalculated and had a prize examination scheduled for 9 a.m. on the morning after the wedding. It was a sign of things to come for Caroline, but as ever, she accepted it stoically and put on a brave front to the maid who came into the hotel room the next morning to find a half-drunk bottle of champagne and an apparently abandoned bride.

Despite periods of pessimism during the examination period, I earned the exhibition alone in two out of three of the final year subjects and shared it in the third and won thirteen out of fifteen special prizes.

CHAPTER 2

It was time now to get on with the practice of medicine. Being aware of my indigent state and new family responsibilities and aware that my intern's salary was at subsistence level, I arranged to do a locum during the vacation. This would be illegal now, as it should be, but it was not too unusual then. I remember vividly my first case as a baby with a rash and trying to work out how to write a prescription for calamine lotion. Shortly after I saw a child with sores in its mouth and, in retrospect, thought of chicken pox, so drove to see the child at home and found some telltale skin vesicles and rapidly revised my diagnosis.

I learnt a lot in those three weeks. My medical course had prepared me for some things, but in other areas, such as sexual counselling, my training had been totally inadequate.

Chapter 3

INTERNSHIP AND CLINICAL TRAINING AT THE ROYAL MELBOURNE HOSPITAL

My first year as a doctor, termed in those days, junior resident medical officer, now known as an intern, were exacting, particularly during the three months in the general medical ward and three months in the general surgical ward. As a single intern looking after on average thirty patients often with complex and multiple diseases, it was often extremely busy.

I undertook my surgical term in the Ackland-Macleish unit. Tom Ackland was a wonderfully committed surgeon, whose particular area of expertise was radical mastectomy for breast cancer, a hugely invasive form of surgery which has been superseded. In contrast to the brutality of the surgery, Tom was very sensitive and caring, characteristics not always found in the surgeons of the time. Scotty Macleish was a precise and meticulous surgeon, who had a particular interest and specialisation in vascular surgery. It was a great unit, but nonetheless, as an intern, I was placed in situations well beyond my competence. Patients died because of fluid and electrolyte problems that today would be dealt with easily. On one night, helped by another intern but with no one more senior, we put a nail through the tibia to allow traction to a fracture of the femur. Another night, I was left alone to try to deal with multiple trauma victims, including a person with a ruptured spleen, while the surgeons were in the theatre.

Times have moved on, but let's not look back with too much nostalgia on a past which was certainly not better than the present.

My medical term was spent in the unit run by John ('Jock'), later Sir John Frew, to whom I will return later, with a delightful gastroenterologist, David Fone, as the outpatient physician. The ward was frenetically busy and dealt with patients with all types of complex medical problems. Jock

CHAPTER 3

had the philosophy that we could deal with everything with minimal help from the newly emerging breed of medical specialists. It was a great learning experience but incredibly demanding. We were rostered on three nights per week, during which we would often get little sleep, and on the nights we were rostered off, we would often not leave until 10 or 11 p.m. Caroline spent many a night in the clinical room of the ward sticking investigation slips into histories. By day, she was working as a psychologist, first at St Nicholas home for intellectually handicapped infants and then at the Children's Court – her income largely supported us. Despite the hours, interns in those days were paid a pittance.

I had an excellent registrar, but despite help from him, we were often put in positions which we were not equipped to deal with.

Some of the problems were of our own making. I particularly remember Christmas Eve, 1967. There was a stoic man, whom I shall call Mr Jones, who had fluid around his lung caused by cancer invading the surface of the lung. I tried to drain the fluid by inserting a broad needle and succeeded in puncturing the lung, causing air to enter the space around the lung above the fluid. I thought that I could solve that by inserting a tube with a sidearm to take the air as well as the fluid away. The net effect was that the air was conveyed from the space around the lung to the tissues under the skin. Because of the distortions caused by the cancer, the air continued to escape from the lung and to track into the tissues under the skin, blowing the hapless Mr Jones up like the Michelin Man. I spent the entire night of Christmas Eve, 1967, puncturing the skin around his face and under his eyes and compressing the tissues to let the air escape, which it did with a hiss. When Jock did his customary ward round on Christmas Day, he found it hugely amusing and brought his consultant colleagues to show them what Richard had done. Ironically and not uniquely, the long-suffering Mr Jones, whom I had so mismanaged, was incredibly grateful for all the attention I had bestowed on him. He required surgery to repair the damage to his diseased lung.

Another traumatic experience was the term in the casualty ward (now more correctly termed the emergency ward). The naïve and inexperienced interns were exposed to the homeless and alcoholics, to the acutely psychiatrically disturbed, the victims of domestic violence and the relentless toll of road accidents. I remember well the night before my scheduled Easter long weekend, for which Caroline and I had planned a camping trip to the Macalister River in Gippsland. I was rostered in casualty overnight on Easter Thursday. My last task before Caroline picked me up on Good Friday morning for us to start our break was to enter an ambulance and declare dead four teenagers killed in a road accident. I drove quite carefully that Easter. It is one of the triumphs of intersectoral research and policy setting that the number of people killed in road accidents is now about one quarter the number of that time, despite a much higher population and very many more vehicles on our roads.

Rostered on three weekday nights and for the full forty-eight hours of one weekend in three meant that there was little opportunity to spend with Caroline in our nearby apartment. We moved a stretcher into the residents' quarters, but the tyrannical housekeeper of the quarters gave us strict instructions that it was forbidden to have guests in your room, even if they were your spouse. Nevertheless, quite a degree of camaraderie developed between the long-suffering spouses of the interns.

By the second year of our residents' program, we were required to differentiate into medical or surgical lines or to leave the hospital for paediatric, obstetric or general practice training. Despite the surgeons and gynaecologists encouraging me to follow their disciplines, I found the variety and intellectual challenge of internal medicine more fitted to my interests and talents. Rotation between different areas of medical specialties and through the professorial unit provided great experience and exposure to talented and committed clinicians. I went through brief phases of thinking I would be a cardiologist, gastroenterologist, haematologist or neurologist.

Third year was spent as a medical registrar. I was chosen for the elite position of registrar to the famous 'Jock' Frew, the chief censor (examiner) of the College of Physicians, soon to become the president of the college, president of the hospital and a knight of the realm. He was legendary because of his clinical experience and acumen, his commitment to daily ward rounds every day of the week, at which he would expect his registrar to be present, and because of a fearsome temper.

For the most part, Jock behaved like a complete gentleman. But three specific events showed that the last part of his reputation had been well earned. As we were nearing the end of a ward round, he said to me that he feared he was losing respect. He then proceeded to tear strips off the admitting officer, a second-year resident, for admitting a 'boarder' (that is a patient belonging to another unit) to our ward. A second time, he did the

CHAPTER 3

same thing to the cardiology registrar for failing to inform him that one of his patients was admitted to the coronary care unit. And the third time, he verbally assaulted a senior radiologist for not performing an X-ray on one of his private patients on the afternoon he had requested it.

On the last occasion, as was customary, I escorted Jock back to his car in the consultants' car park. Nothing was said, but he must have sensed my disapproval. As he stepped into his car he said, 'You are right, Richard, I shouldn't do that sort of thing. My wife tells me that too'. At least some insight, but it was also clear that he had carefully orchestrated at least some of the events to ensure that he preserved his reputation and people did what he wanted.

Unlike the current regimented system, physician training consisted of acquiring the appropriate blend of posts within a teaching hospital and then sitting the Royal Australasian College of Physicians examination a minimum of three years after graduation. I undertook my examination at the earliest time I was able, at the beginning of my fourth year, and to my relief I passed the written and clinical examinations (and was told at the traditional sherry party for successful candidates that I received the highest marks for the examination in the country).

At that stage, I was still intent on pursuing a career partly in private and partly working as a consultant in a hospital following the pattern of the role models to whom I had been most exposed, such as Jock Frew, David Fone, Ken Fairley, Margaret Henderson and other fine physicians. I wanted to be a general physician with a particular interest and expertise in a specialist area, again following the pattern of what I had seen. So what was to be the area of particular interest?

I had experienced a variety of medical specialties up to that time and several had appealed to me. But I was also broadly interested in the whole person and all the body systems and did not wish to confine myself too narrowly. One area where I had had no particular experience was endocrinology and I had given it no serious consideration. I was therefore surprised when the director of diabetes and endocrinology, Ian ('Skip') Martin, suggested that I might like to take the position grandly titled Assistant Endocrinologist, although it was effectively equivalent to registrar in diabetes and endocrinology. On reflection, endocrinology did bring in the entire body through the chemical messengers that controlled all the organ systems, and diabetes, with its complications, similarly impacted the whole body. In addition, exciting breakthroughs were occurring, with new hormones being discovered through radioimmunoassays able to detect tiny quantities of circulating hormones.

It was a fortunate decision, one of a small number which have had a decisive impact on the direction my career has taken. Skip Martin was an amazing character. Although only employed six-tenths by the hospital, with the remainder of his time in private practice, his insatiable curiosity had led him to develop a variety of research programs. These ranged from defining a relationship between resistance to the blood sugar lowering effects of insulin and the development of the complications of diabetes, through to the role of the recently described long-acting thyroid stimulator (LATS), now known as thyroid stimulating immunoglobulin (TSI), in the recurrence of thyrotoxicosis after treatment and the description of a new type of diabetes in the highlands of Papua New Guinea.

I had never previously contemplated research and without Skip's influence I may well never have done so. He introduced me to some fat mice from New Zealand, which were in the adjoining Walter and Eliza Hall Institute. They had been brought there from the University of Otago, because they were related to other New Zealand mice which had evidence of antibodies to their own tissues. The fat mice (New Zealand Obese or NZO mice) did not show evidence of autoantibodies, but Skip suggested I should study their hormones to see if they could be a model for obesity and diabetes in humans.

As many medical graduates had found before me, embarking on laboratory-based medical research is a deflating experience. Having been a hospital registrar with considerable standing in the ward and confidence in managing sick patients, I was suddenly exposed to an environment where I had only theoretical knowledge and was completely devoid of practical skills or experience. I remember particularly a painful experience of being abused by an eighteen-year-old laboratory technician for not using the centrifuge correctly.

My first trial experience at presenting a scientific paper was a similarly humiliating experience. Skip Martin had generously offered me the opportunity to present a paper to the annual meeting of the Endocrine Society of Australia, which largely reflected his work on the ability of the LATS level to predict the liability of relapse in thyrotoxicosis after remission following radioactive iodine treatment. I gave a practice presentation to the Department of Medicine. At the conclusion, Dick Lovell said simply, 'That was dreadful, Richard!'

CHAPTER 3

I had read the presentation rapidly and it was generally unintelligible. Chastened, I had another go a few days later, basically talking to the slides and slowing down considerably. I was gratified by words of praise, and the subsequent presentation to the Endocrine Society went well. To this day, my presentations are generally better, if a little unpredictable, if I ad-lib them rather than read them.

After those setbacks, I muddled through and set up radioimmunoassays for mouse insulin and growth hormone. I found that the NZO mouse was an excellent model for type 2 diabetes in humans. They had high basal insulin levels and insulin resistance combined with a defective insulin response to glucose and a number of other agents. In contrast, they had a hugely enhanced release of insulin in response to the amino acid arginine. This meant that their pancreases were not 'exhausted' or depleted of insulin, but that there was a disorder in the glucose-signalling mechanism. My second paper was published in *Nature New Biology*, one of the Nature stable of journals, the elite of scientific publications, and two others were in *Diabetes* and in *Diabetologia*, the leading diabetes journals in the USA and Europe respectively.

I was able to write up this research into a dissertation which complemented an examination taken for the first part of the doctor of medicine degree to complete the requirements for that qualification. I was still intending at that stage to have a largely clinical career, but a research doctorate would be very helpful in gaining a consultant's post at a leading teaching hospital such as the Royal Melbourne, the limit of my ambition at that stage.

Apart from this introduction to research, the two and a half years I spent as the assistant endocrinologist was also very rewarding from the point of view of learning the essentials of clinical endocrinology and diabetes. It was an exciting time in endocrinology, as prolactin had just been discovered as a new hormone secreted by the pituitary and the product of many pituitary tumours previously thought to be inactive. Shortly after, a drug called bromocriptine was found not only to markedly reduce prolactin production from these tumours, allowing many infertile women to conceive, but also to dramatically reduce the size of the tumours, sometimes restoring vision that had been impaired by the expanding tumour compressing the optic nerve. Skip Martin was a wonderful role model, clearly loving his work and having a genuine interest in and rapport with his patients.

The question then arose: What next? Until a decade or so before, it had been almost mandatory for a physician or surgeon wishing to rise to the top of his or her profession to go to the UK for further clinical training and to complete a membership examination of one of the Royal Colleges in England or Scotland. It was now clear, however, that the Australian MRACP was more demanding than the British college examinations, so it was no longer necessary to do clinical training in the UK. However, it was still felt appropriate that one should have 'overseas experience'.

Having not followed the traditional academic or research route, I was not eligible for the prestigious and generous C.J. Martin Fellowships of the National Health and Medical Research Council, so I was fortunate instead to be awarded a full year of funding (albeit parsimonious) in the form of a Churchill Fellowship. The most exacting part of the process of gaining the Churchill Fellowship was the interview by a large panel chaired by a justice of the Supreme Court. He knew my barrister brother, John, and said that didn't I think that it was silly to contemplate a life in research, as I would not earn nearly as much money as John. I was able to reply that I didn't spend as much either and that seemed to satisfy him and the panel sufficiently to be awarded the fellowship.

I had received some advice from colleagues in the Department of Medicine at the Royal Melbourne Hospital and resolved to work with Professor Iain MacIntyre at the Royal Postgraduate Medical School at Hammersmith Hospital. So, with two young children and a still biddable wife in tow, we set out on a Boeing 707 for the UK.

Chapter 4

LONDON

Our arrival in London in August 1972 was not auspicious. We were tired after a thirty-three-hour flight, which included, as the kangaroo route then did, five stops. We had also discovered our eighteen-month-old daughter, Fiona, was one of the 10 per cent of infants in whom the sedative Vallergan had a paradoxical excitatory effect. So, much of the thirty-three hours had been spent with Fiona joyously pulling herself up in her bassinet and saying hello – little sleep, but at least she was happy.

Arriving at Heathrow in the early morning, we were asked for our health certificates. No one had told us we needed these, so we were herded into a vast hall which seemed to contain about 1000 people, almost exclusively apparently from the Indian subcontinent. A white doctor came into the hall, looked at us and said that we looked healthy enough, so we could leave with the appropriate clearance. I was appalled by this obvious racism and was about to protest, when a look from Caroline told me that if I wished to survive the day, I should accept the kindly offered favour.

Temporary accommodation had been organised in Middlesex Hospital residential quarters in Lancaster Gate. The plan was for us to spend a week there before moving into our permanent accommodation. This was to be a house in North Wembley, rented from a registrar at the Hammersmith Hospital who was to spend a year or so working in India. Somewhat foolishly, while tired and jet-lagged, we decided to have a look at the house on the afternoon of our arrival. We tackled the Bakerloo Line and British Rail to travel out to North Wembley and were somewhat dismayed to see a very unpretentious semi-detached house with an orange door and overgrown garden.

'I am not going to live there', Caroline declared. Deflated, we returned to Lancaster Gate and spent the next couple of days looking. An advertisement for a two-bedroom flat overlooking Hampstead Heath sounded more appealing – but it was minute, Hampstead Heath was a distant glimpse and it cost £30, rather than £20, per week – and our scholarship was only going to deliver £56 per week before tax.

So chastened, we moved into the house with the orange door. It served our needs well, albeit in modest rather than luxurious surroundings, and Caroline once more showed her capacity to adapt. Our older daughter, Sarah, went to the local preschool centre and we joined the babysitting club. Our next-door neighbour, an elderly widow, took pity on us and insisted on looking after the children for one day a week while Caroline was able to sample some of the delights of London.

Iain MacIntyre and his delightful Scottish wife, Mabs, went out of their way to help us to settle in. Shortly after we arrived, they invited us to their house in Fulham for dinner. Caroline asked Mabs where she did her weekly shopping and Mabs gave the particularly helpful advice that she simply got into a taxi and went to Harrods food hall in nearby Knightsbridge. Caroline found that Sainsbury's in Wembley was a bit more practical on my miserable scholarship. Iain plied us with wine and we left to try to navigate back to North Wembley in a slightly tipsy state (we didn't know at that time that drinking and driving meant we were bloody idiots).

We had bought a twelve-year-old Morris Oxford. I had plotted a route home, but it entailed doing a forbidden turn into Fulham Palace Road. Shortly after we did this, I was pulled up by a policeman. With the dual sins of having drunk too much and having done an illegal turn, I could see dire consequences ahead. It got worse when the policeman asked me to get out of the car. I did so and he pointed to the beam of my headlights. He said they were pointing incorrectly. He then explained how I could fix them with a screwdriver or even a knitting needle but then said very helpfully that I didn't need them anyway – the parking lights were plenty. He wished me well and we were on our way. That was our introduction to the legendary politeness of the British constabulary! I fear that with first the IRA terrorism and more recently Muslim jihadists, their role and attitude may have altered substantially since then.

That episode of generosity and hospitality was typical of the MacIntyres – they invited us as their guests to the Hurlingham Club Ball and other social gatherings – more than a junior researcher from the colonies could have expected of the venerable head of the department. It certainly gave us some

CHAPTER 4

insights into how the less impoverished elements of London society were able to entertain themselves.

I was to work in the recently emerged 'hot area', the metabolism of vitamin D. In the last couple of years, it had been found that far from being a vitamin in the true sense, vitamin D was largely synthesised in skin under the influence of sunlight, and then it was activated by a two-step process, first in the liver, which converted it to its major circulating form, 25-hydroxy vitamin D, and then in the kidney to the biologically active form, 1,25-dihydroxy vitamin D. This last step appeared to be finely regulated according to the biological need for calcium.

Iain suggested that I work on the regulation of this metabolic process in the kidney and referred to some recent work where renal tubules from vitamin D-deficient chicks served as a model in which to study this. He also suggested that since it had recently been proposed by Hector De Luca and his colleagues in Wisconsin that the parathyroid hormone was the key factor determining the response to low calcium levels, we should see the effect of removal of the parathyroid glands in rats on the response to a low calcium diet. Macintyre's group had recently published a very controversial article in the *Lancet* suggesting that far from being the mediator of the response to low calcium levels, the injection of parathyroid hormone in rats actually suppressed the formation of the active metabolite, the reverse effect compared to that expected from De Luca's work.

So with colleagues, we commenced work on preparing vitamin D-deficient chicks and rats, learning how to remove parathyroids from rats (they are tiny, so they are removed together with the thyroid gland in which they are embedded) and digesting the tubules from chick kidneys and learning how to incubate them so that they could be tested for their ability to convert the inactive precursor, 25-hydroxy vitamin D to the active form. The techniques were quite similar to those I had earlier used to isolate pancreatic islets from mice.

Not long after starting this work, Iain suggested that it would be valuable for me and colleagues from his laboratory to go to Vienna to attend a big European calcium conference. Caroline and I thought it would be a great opportunity to see a bit of Europe, so we set off in our newly acquired Morris Oxford with our two children in the back seat. Getting to Dover to catch the ferry was a saga in its own right. The car wouldn't start, it boiled at least four times on the road to Dover and at that time the so-called South Circular was really a series of poorly connected and highly congested suburban streets. Despite having allowed what we thought was an extravagant amount of time, we were the last car to be allowed on the ferry, just as the car bridge was about to be drawn up.

We made our way to Vienna with a series of experiences in 'pensions' and a real taste of the Rhine Valley and Germany. Unfortunately, accommodation was impossible to find in Vienna. At one accommodation centre for tourists we encountered a young woman who told us she knew a place where we could stay. It turned out, it seemed, to be some form of refuge for homeless and alcoholic men, and we spent a noisy and uncomfortable night in the smelly and inhospitable place. It was made worse in the morning when we discovered that Caroline's new Jaeger coat (our one extravagance since arriving in London) had been stolen from the car. We consoled ourselves with breakfast in a famous hotel served by gentlemen in dinner jackets, wiser and poorer than before.

Things looked up from there. We were then able to book into a venerable old pension that had previously been a grand home, with a wide stone staircase. I attended the meeting and then the conference dinner at a 'heuriger' or launch of the new vintage of wine – another occasion where I was a bloody idiot and made it home only by following the tram lines on the assumption that they would lead to the centre of the city, where we thought we might find our pension. Caroline and I share a memory of swaying up the stone staircase and being greeted by a very disapproving Viennese babysitter.

After my first introduction to an international meeting, we made our way through the Dolomites and north Italy to Chamonix. The car was clearly struggling and it was frequently necessary to pour cold water into its radiator when it boiled. It finally gave up the ghost on the alpine road between Chamonix and Geneva, where I was due to give a talk about my work on the NZO mice to the famed Institut Biochimie Clinique with its legendary director, Albert Renold. After walking back to a dubious service station to get help and being perilously towed back to Chamonix for repairs, we hired a car and drove quickly to Geneva just in time to be picked up by Professor Renold. After delivering my seminar, I was driven back to the hotel to discover my hired car had been towed away, as it was illegally parked – I could not interpret the sign and in any case I had no time to park it legally. Eventually I was able to recover the car (leaving my watch in lieu of the fine) and had a great night enjoying the hospitality of the institute. I was invited to spend

CHAPTER 4

two years there after finishing in London, and I regret that my eagerness to accept a job offered to me from Australia led to me not taking up this offer.

The first few months of my work in London went well. With my colleague Seamus MacCauley, we managed to get renal tubules from vitamin D-deficient chicks to convert the inactive circulating form of vitamin D to its active product and to show that this was a regulated conversion dependent in a complex way on the level of calcium and hormones and that the active form of vitamin D fed back to inhibit the conversion.

As I had found with my rat growth hormone assays in Melbourne, rapid early progress is often followed by a period of frustration. For six months, nothing worked. The technical details are not important at this time, but the oft-stated comment that you learn much more by trying to work out why an experiment is not working rather than by blindly and successfully following a technique developed by others was once again demonstrated to us. Eventually, we sorted it out and things progressed once more.

Our experiments in rats were also successful. We showed that parathyroid hormone was not essential for rats to respond to dietary challenges by increasing conversion of the inactive form of vitamin D to its active form, a controversial issue at the time.

I also learnt a little about how the British medical journal publishing occurred, at least in that era. MacIntyre was excited about our rat results and thought that it would be good for them to be published in a high-profile journal. So he rang the editor of the *Lancet*, told him that these results were really exciting and that the *Lancet* should publish them. I was invited to have afternoon tea with the editor. We had a pleasant discussion about the findings and their significance and the article appeared in the pages of the revered *Lancet* about four weeks later. Gratifying, but it was also a discomforting insight into how far away we were from the seat of power when we plaintively sent our articles off to unknown and distant editorial boards from our home base in Australia.

An illustration of the vigour of scientific debate came at a symposium held at Hammersmith and hosted by Iain MacIntyre. This was part of a series of such symposia held at two-year intervals, initially focusing on calcitonin, a newly discovered hormone which lowered calcium levels. The MacIntyre laboratory had made seminal contributions to understanding its physiology. The conference had been broadened to calcium metabolism and bones more generally. Hector De Luca from the University of Wisconsin in Madison had provided evidence that parathyroid hormone mediated the increased formation of the active form of vitamin D in low calcium conditions, whereas MacIntyre's lab had found the effect of injected parathyroid hormone to be inhibitory rather than stimulatory. MacIntyre, with his Scottish delight in controversy, made provocative statements inflaming what had already become a heated debate to the obvious discomfort of De Luca, an invited guest.

At dinner that evening I had the privilege of sitting next to a revered and senior figure, who was head of endocrinology and professor of medicine at Massachusetts General Hospital. He lamented the provocative nature of the presentation. He contrasted it with his own dignified response to the controversy around the structure of parathyroid hormone. He then went on to say that 'someone had set out to destroy him and his career, but he would get him by the balls and show him'. Paranoia and aggression were alive and well despite his encouragement of dignity under fire. I preferred the more open, albeit provocative, Scottish approach of the good-natured MacIntyre to the covert and smouldering hostility expressed on the other side of the Atlantic.

After one year in London, it was suggested that I should go and present my findings at a calcium and bone meeting held in Rochester, Minnesota, the home of the Mayo Clinic. I extended my trip for a total period of six weeks to allow me to visit a number of laboratories around the country, concentrating not only on those dealing with vitamin D and calcium, but also visiting research groups and institutes doing diabetes research so that I could keep up with that field as well.

At the conference in Rochester, I experienced a little of the cut and thrust of the scientific world in the United States. A pugnacious senior professor with an established extensive reputation in calcium metabolism questioned me after my presentation, in which I showed an extensive array of results of experiments using the renal tubules indicating that they readily converted the vitamin to its active form and that a variety of factors influenced the rate of this conversion. He said that he had tried thirty-five times to get renal tubules to do this conversion but that they had completely failed to do so. I was grateful when someone in the audience called out, 'You should have tried a thirty-sixth time, Lou'.

The rest of my trip was very rewarding. Several celebrities in diabetes research were incredibly hospitable and helpful – people like George Cahill,

CHAPTER 4

who was the director of the Joslin Clinic in Boston, the world's leading centre for diabetes research and clinical care, Jesse Roth, the director of the diabetes, metabolism and renal section of the National Institutes of Health in Bethesda, Paul Lacy in St Louis, a pioneer in pancreatic islet transplantation and Doug Coleman at Bar Harbor in Maine, who did pioneering work using mouse models for diabetes. I had a Shabbat dinner with Saul Genuth in Cleveland and stayed with Barbara and Doug Coleman in Bar Harbor after taking the Greyhound bus there. I stayed with my former Trinity tutor Ian McKenzie and fellow Australians Mary and Geoff Tregear in Boston, who were minding a large house in Boston while its owner was on holiday. I also saw Hugh Niall in Boston, who with Geoff Tregear was working on the structure of parathyroid hormone at Massachusetts General Hospital and in the midst of a heated and public controversy with Brian Brewer at NIH about a disputed four amino acids in the structure. These Australians were having a huge impact on international science.

My experience in St Louis was particularly helpful. The transplantation of pancreatic islets was emerging as one of the most exciting fields of research in diabetes with the prospect of curing type 1, or insulin-dependent diabetes, the form which most often has its onset in young people. I was contemplating this as an area of research, but my experience in St Louis and later experience with human islets in Uppsala convinced me that the supply and isolation of islets and immunosuppression to prevent their rejection were formidable problems for which my background did not particularly equip me. I decided that it was probably not a field I should personally pursue.

After a few months in London, I decided to enrol in a PhD. Although I had a research doctorate already from the University of Melbourne, it did seem like a golden opportunity to extend my work in London so that I could submit it for a PhD through the University of London. MacIntyre arranged a Medical Research Council fellowship for my second year. Finances were still a problem, as we had to move to another house that would cost £120 per month instead of the previous £80 per month. This was almost half my fellowship before tax, so we had little money to spare. By and large, the research progressed well and I had completed the first draft of my thesis about three months before the two-year minimum time for submission.

It was before the days of widespread use of word processors and computers. The first draft was handwritten, and the typist, who was a neighbour and a member of our babysitting club, was asked to type an original with a carbon copy, which would be submitted to MacIntyre as my supervisor. Caroline had produced our third daughter, Kate, a month earlier.

We were due to go out to dinner with an Australian friend on the evening that Caroline was picking up the thesis. She was unusually quiet when I arrived home. I helped our oldest daughter Sarah with her bath when somewhat unexpectedly she said, 'Daddy, you will never guess what happened to your thesis today. It was spread page by page all the way between North Wembley and Wembley.' She was parroting what she had heard from her distraught mother that afternoon as she talked to some friends on the phone.

It turned out that when Caroline picked up the original and the two typed copies of the thesis, the typist's mother had asked to see the baby. Caroline produced the basket containing Kate from the back seat, swelled with pride at the 'oohs and ahhs' about how beautiful the baby was, replaced the basket and drove off. She said that she then had a sudden feeling of alarm and asked Sarah whether Daddy's thesis was on the seat beside her. It was not. It had been put on the roof of the car when the basket was taken from the back seat and Caroline had driven off with it there. It was a still day, so the thesis came off page by page as Caroline drove to the supermarket in Wembley to do her shopping. When she realised what had happened, she retraced her steps and found a pack of boy scouts, whom she enlisted to find as much of the thesis as they could. Being tidy, several of the householders had already put pages in their bins and other pages had been run over by trucks or bicycles. With much effort, either one of the typed copies or the original was found for all but three pages, which I rewrote. That event aged us both prematurely, but the fact that our marriage survived unscathed suggested that we were wed for the long haul.

My two years in London had been very rewarding from the research point of view, as the PhD produced six publications, including one in *Lancet* and one in *Nature*. The latter described the interaction between a nuclear action of 1,25-dihydroxyvitamin D and calcium levels in the feedback regulation of vitamin D metabolism in the kidney.

Living in London was also a wonderful experience, despite our penury. We were able to watch Nureyev and Fonteyn dance and listen to the Royal Opera Company at Covent Garden from seats in the 'gods'. We had wonderful holiday excursions to Cornwall, Scotland, Wales and Paris.

CHAPTER 4

The research experience may have come at a cost. Occupational health and safety was not well developed at that time. We had a room full of chromatography columns attached to multiple circular fraction collectors, which allowed us to run something like fifteen columns at a time. The eluting fluid was a mixture of organic solvents designed to separate the different vitamin D compounds. The room was poorly ventilated and full of fumes. I and Iain MacIntyre both developed bladder cancers twenty-five or so years later. Exposure to the organic solvents may have contributed.

At first I attempted to keep some clinical involvement going by attending outpatients and ward rounds in diabetes and endocrinology. But having sat as a passive observer watching the consultant perform diabetes care to a lower standard than that to which I had been accustomed in Australia and being told that there was such demand to be a clinical observer, we would be placed on a 'rota', I decided to forego the privilege. I kept my clinical interests satisfied to some extent by attending the weekly grand round. These were theatrical productions with many of the recognised world experts on the cases being present in the audience, either because they were members of the illustrious Hammersmith staff or as visitors passing through.

I handed in the thesis in the minimum time of two years. The practice at the University of London was to require the candidate to present in person for an oral defence of the thesis with the examiners. A period of three months was required between submission and the defence. We took advantage of this time to spend three months driving through Europe. This had the added advantage of allowing us to take our new car out of England for three months and to then ship it back to Australia duty-free. In retrospect, I am not sure how we managed to drive around Holland, Germany, Scandinavia, Switzerland and France for three months with a seven-month-old baby, two children aged six and three and all the supporting paraphernalia in a relatively small sedan car. We stayed in pensions, except for a few days in university accommodation in Aarhus in Denmark and one week in Umea and three weeks in Uppsala. I visited a number of laboratories in this time, made a number of new contacts, learnt some new techniques and we also saw a great deal of Europe.

One experience I was grateful for occurred during a three-week sojourn in Claes Hellerstrom's and Arne Andersson's laboratory in Uppsala. We spent a night trying to prepare human pancreatic islets for transplantation from a recent donor pancreas. This was an extremely difficult process. The human pancreas was much more fibrous than that of the mice and rats that I had been used to and the islets were very difficult to isolate free of the other pancreatic tissue. This experience reinforced my decision not to devote my career to human pancreatic islet transplantation.

It was about thirty years before a group in Edmonton Canada developed a viable process to prepare islets and to immunosuppress the recipient sufficiently to allow successful clinical islet transplantation. Ironically, recently I was on the board of the Australian Islet Transplantation Program, a successful program jointly funded by the National Health and Medical Research Council of Australia and the Juvenile Diabetes Foundation International. The process remains too demanding for routine clinical use, but it is gratifying that it has progressed to the stage where it is transforming the lives of the small number of people with diabetes where other therapies have failed and who are suitable for islet transplantation.

At the end of the continental European odyssey, we returned to London for me to 'defend' my thesis, which I managed to do to the satisfaction of my examiners. It was then time to return to Australia and to start a proper job!

Chapter 5

THE SENIOR MEDICAL STAFF OF THE ROYAL MELBOURNE HOSPITAL

I returned to Melbourne in November 1974 to be located geographically full-time at the Royal Melbourne Hospital. I had dual appointments. One was to the newly created post of physician to the endocrine laboratory. In this role I would be responsible for the assay activities of the endocrine laboratory with its expanding number of radioimmunoassays. I was also expected to undertake research and supervise research training and was involved in clinical and teaching activities both in outpatient clinics and with ward patients and referrals. My second appointment was as physician to outpatients in what became the Fairley-Larkins Unit. At that time, the custom was that the five general medical units each had an inpatient physician and a more junior outpatient physician. Once appointed to an outpatient physician position, a young physician became a member of the senior medical staff and had an assured future as a consultant physician.

In most cases, the physicians (both inpatient and outpatient) serving the general medical units were very much part-time in the hospital and spent the majority of their time in private practice. One or two other physicians with a primary specialist role in the hospital had been appointed to general medical units, a trend which was to increase over time. The hierarchical relationship of the inpatient versus outpatient appointments and the differentiation between senior and other medical staff were not to survive the more egalitarian time of the 1980s, but it was alive and well then.

I learnt a great deal in my general medical unit and enjoyed it immensely. Ken Fairley is a remarkable man with incredible energy, clinical experience and acumen and an infectious curiosity. This had led him as a clinician to make some important research observations of great clinical significance.

An example was his description of the different morphology of red blood cells in the urine originating from the kidneys versus those coming from the ureters, bladder or urethra. This allowed identification of the likely site of bleeding in cases of blood in the urine merely from microscopic examination of the urine, which in turn determined the subsequent diagnostic approach.

We always finished our joint ward rounds with a visit to pathology to examine specimens at first hand – often with the aid of his equally talented wife, Priscilla Kincaid-Smith. They were both wonderful role models for budding clinician-scientists.

One aspect of their life that I would not recommend anyone should try to replicate was their weekends. They had a property at Apollo Bay, an idyllic location about three hours by car from Melbourne. They had arrangements for young physicians to look after their patients over the weekend and went there just about every week. They lived with their twin boys and daughter in a caravan, old railway carriage or shed for many years before their house was complete. They farmed like dervishes. No challenge, physical or agricultural, was too great. Ken drove bulldozers; Priscilla drove the tractor and rode bareback.

They were also very generous hosts and invited Caroline and me there for a weekend. We were put to work. I was asked to drive a tractor down a sheer hill, dragging a harrow behind. The harrow was the only thing stopping the tractor getting out of control and even then, because of bare rock in the middle of the paddock, it careered down over that section. I had memories of my days in Corryong, where my father was too frequently called out to tractor accidents where the farmer had rolled the tractor on himself and died. Caroline rode a horse to herd cattle. We flew in a small plane, metres above the crops, sat on the front bonnet of a 'ute' to shoot rabbits and generally had an exhilarating but perilous time. Ken had a number of accidents, including one in a bulldozer that he rolled and only survived because he rolled down the slope a bit faster than the bulldozer. One of his registrars shortly after broke her arm in an accident on the farm.

They remain, in their eighties, a wonderful, talented and larger than life couple living life to the full. Priscilla was a real trailblazer for academic and medical women, becoming the first female professor at the University of Melbourne when she was appointed to a personal chair and the first female president of the Royal Australasian College of Physicians. She built a world-class nephrology unit at the Royal Melbourne Hospital and was

CHAPTER 5

also active in the Australian Medical Association, where she became chair of its National Assembly.

My time in the endocrinology laboratory was also rewarding. I had some time for research, which was partly clinical and partly laboratory-based, and I supervised my first two PhD students. I continued my interest in vitamin D and was also able to resume studies of insulin release in the NZO mouse. One of my PhD students, Paula Heyma, used the renal tubule model I had been working on in London to study the newly described phenomenon of conversion of thyroxine to a more active product, triiodothyronine. I was discovering a recurrent theme in my research career: lessons and techniques learnt from the study of one system could often be applied profitably to another; work spanning the breadth of different systems, as well as the breadth from clinical work through to basic research, allowed unique perspectives.

My hospital clinical work was complemented by a small private practice. It was based in the private consulting rooms at the hospital. I initially did this on Saturday mornings, but as it grew, I later devoted a half day during the week to it. The very personal relationship with individual patients and the sense of individual responsibility was something that I valued and I continued the half day until I moved to Monash as vice-chancellor in 2003. Telling my long-term patients at that time that I was ceasing practice caused me much regret. I had known some for almost thirty years and, although only seeing them once or twice a year, felt I had been through their life and family traumas as they grew from teenagers to mature adults and parents. It is a privilege of medical practice and it especially applies to general practice and specialist practice involving chronic diseases such as diabetes mellitus.

I was also fully involved in education. I found I greatly enjoyed the combination of clinical duties and teaching in both general medicine and endocrinology and research, both laboratory-based and clinical. I started to think that I could preserve this balance better in an academic position in a university clinical department than in a combination of hospital positions. I discussed this with Dick Lovell, who was very supportive but pointed out that there were no vacant positions in the department of medicine at the Royal Melbourne Hospital at that time.

Coincidentally, Jack Martin had decided to return from his chair of chemical pathology at the University of Sheffield to become the foundation professor of medicine at the Repatriation General Hospital, Heidelberg. This was a branch of the Austin Hospital department of medicine of the

NEW TRICKS

University of Melbourne, which was headed by Austin Doyle. I had come across Jack Martin on a number of previous occasions. He had been a demonstrator in our biochemistry practical classes when I was a medical student, and he had been a senior lecturer (then quaintly termed second assistant) in Dick Lovell's department of medicine at the Royal Melbourne Hospital when I was a resident in that unit. More recently, he had come over to Hammersmith to undertake a sabbatical with Iain MacIntyre while I was doing my PhD there. Caroline and I became quite close to Jack and his delightful wife, Christine, and I was enormously impressed by Jack's passion for research.

Jack was recruited from Hammersmith to his chair at Sheffield and was there for about three years before taking up the chair at the Repatriation General Hospital. He offered me the position grandly titled first assistant (equivalent to associate professor) and because of my desire to increase my research involvement I decided to accept.

This caused quite a commotion at the Royal Melbourne Hospital. No one ever voluntarily left a position on its senior medical staff before the compulsory retirement age, unless provoked to do so by a run-in with the management or professional colleagues. When I told the president of the hospital, Sir John ('Jock') Frew, that I was leaving, he was outraged. I had been both an intern and registrar in his unit and he had been hugely supportive. He gave me quite a dressing down.

'The trouble with you, Richard, is that you are immature. If you ever wanted to be professor of medicine at the Royal Melbourne Hospital, you have laid the way wide open for 'X' (a professional colleague at the hospital and an outstanding researcher).

For once, despite the tirade, I managed to say, 'That is excellent, because X would be a very good professor of medicine.' As it turned out, X did not wish to be a professor of medicine and instead had a very distinguished career in research.

This episode highlighted the prevailing thinking at the time. There could be nothing to compare with a senior post at the Royal Melbourne Hospital and anyone contemplating leaving it would be committing professional suicide. Moreover, the only academic position anyone could reasonably aspire to should be at the Royal Melbourne Hospital and in the University of Melbourne. It is ironic that I did return to be a professor of medicine at the hospital, although that was not a specific ambition at the time. I

CHAPTER 5

do not believe that my research achievements would have allowed that appointment if I had not had the courage to leave the hospital.

Times have changed since then and it is recognised that professional exchange between hospitals, universities and even countries is beneficial to all involved. Certainly, for me, the decision to make that move was enormously important and determined to a large extent my subsequent career path, although I did not know it at the time.

My decision at that time was not an easy one for Caroline. After years of living on a pittance as a resident medical officer and PhD student, I finally had a proper job with a good salary. Moreover, it was prestigious and with an assured future. The Repatriation General Hospital was a respected institution from its service to war veterans but was rundown and had many demountable wards and offices which should have been replaced years before. Heidelberg at that time was an outer suburb of lower middle-class socio-economic status. Moreover, my salary was considerably less than I had been receiving at the Royal Melbourne. So to her it must have seemed like a crazy move, completely ignoring the needs of our young family.

As so often before and since, after a period of moderately intense discussion, Caroline said something along the lines of, 'If that is what you really want, go ahead'.

Chapter 6

THE REPATRIATION GENERAL HOSPITAL HEIDELBERG

Life at 'Repat' was different. The patients in 1978 were still mostly ex-servicemen or their widows, although the hospital was attempting to open its doors to the general community. At that stage, it was still directly funded by the commonwealth in contrast to the state-funded public hospitals, such as the Royal Melbourne, the Austin, St Vincent's, the Alfred and Prince Henry's. This led to resistance to the idea that non-veterans be treated at Repat, as commonwealth rather than state funds would need to be used. A few years later, the commonwealth and states came to an agreement allowing the states to fund and administer the repatriation hospitals, allowing much greater integration of services and less paranoia about the treatment of non-veteran patients at the hospital.

Although there had previously been a small section of the Austin department of medicine located at the Repat, with a small laboratory in the old morgue, the creation of the chair and supporting positions, including my first assistant position, greatly expanded it and led to the need for more laboratory and office space. This was gradually provided, although in a piecemeal and makeshift manner, so that the early years were somewhat fraught with many moves of offices and renovations to allow sufficient laboratory space.

Despite the frustrations, it was a wonderful time, extremely rewarding professionally. I was soon asked to direct the endocrinology service as well as to continue a significant general medical responsibility. I ran the diagnostic endocrinology laboratory and conducted postgraduate endocrinology tutorials and clinical medical tutorials for the registrars from the Austin and the Repat who were undertaking their physician training before sitting the feared fellowship examination of the Royal Australasian College of Physicians examinations.

CHAPTER 6

My research prospered as I learnt a lot from Jack Martin, particularly about calcium and bone metabolism and about the relatively new field of prostaglandins and leukotrienes. These were ubiquitous chemicals made from fatty acids in blood cells, the lining cells of blood vessels and in most other tissues. They had many actions which were in the process of being defined. Applying assays for these substances in people and animal models for diabetes and attempting to determine their role in diabetic complications and in insulin release was an exciting new field for me.

In addition, a very bright young woman who had undertaken her master of science with John Court at the Royal Children's Hospital sought me out and asked me to supervise her PhD. Her name was Marjorie Dunlop and it was the beginning of a scientific association that lasted twenty-five years. Marjorie read scientific publications prodigiously, had 'green fingers' in the laboratory and a wonderfully lateral and creative mind. She also had a quirky sense of humour, as illustrated by the Gary Larson cartoon I referred to in the Preface, which kept us all positive and excited by what we were doing. I owe a great deal to her and know that I could have achieved only a fraction of what I was fortunate to achieve in science without the partnership that I formed with her. Her PhD was on the effect of caffeine on growth and insulin release in rat foetuses. This led her to study the effect of caffeine on calcium fluxes in cells, a recurrent theme which I had first broached when studying vitamin D metabolism in London but which Marjorie took to new levels. Marjorie later moved to work full-time with me and, as my clinical work, teaching, administrative and external duties took more time, became functionally the head of our laboratory.

A notable event during my time at Heidelberg was the sabbatical period undertaken in Jack Martin's laboratory by my PhD supervisor and Jack's long-term friend and collaborator, Iain MacIntyre from Hammersmith. Although he spent quite a lot of his time giving talks and travelling, he added an additional element of excitement to the department. It had been a long time since he had physically worked in a laboratory himself, so it was somewhat theatrical and unpredictable when he donned his white coat to do an experiment. All the laboratory staff were suborned to find him things and to work the various instruments and it slowed everything down immensely. Balanced against this was his extremely active and curious mind, which never stopped enthusiastically proposing new hypotheses. He worked with a colleague in our lab, John Eisman, on 1,25-dihydroxyvitamin D receptors in breast and other cancers, an exciting new area of research where Eisman had made major contributions.

The head of the combined Austin and Repatriation department of medicine was Professor Austin Doyle, one of the real characters of Australian medicine.

Highly intelligent, he came originally from Britain via the University of Otago. He had made major contributions to hypertension research. He had originally joined the department of medicine at the Royal Melbourne Hospital as first assistant and reader. He then became the foundation professor of medicine for the new University of Melbourne department of medicine established at the Austin Hospital in the late 1960s. It soon seemed that the hospital had been named after him.

Unlike the situation at the Royal Melbourne Hospital and in other Australian teaching hospitals at the time, at the Austin Hospital the professors of medicine and surgery were made head of their respective hospital divisions, giving a central role to the university in the development and delivery of the clinical services of the hospital. This was closer to the North American model of university hospitals. Austin proceeded to attract an outstanding group of young physician scientists to the new Austin department of medicine, which rapidly became one of the strongest in the country.

Austin Doyle was an unusual-looking man. He had a pot belly, large and protuberant lips and bulging eyes. He had a quick and acerbic wit. He was feared by students and residents who were not adequately prepared, but he was immensely loyal to those he respected and the respect and loyalty were reciprocated by those who worked with him and knew him well. He smoked like a chimney.

Shortly before leaving at the end of six months sabbatical, the MacIntyres held a farewell party in their flat. As was his wont at that time, Austin Doyle had imbibed more than he should have. His features became more prominent, his gait unsteady. He was talking to Mabs, who, unaccustomed to Austin's behaviour, backed away cautiously against the arm of a couch. Austin lost his balance and lurched forwards, and Mabs fell backwards over the arm of the couch, her legs splayed with Austin between them. He lumbered home sheepishly, escorted by his long-suffering and delightful wife, Jill.

CHAPTER 6

Doyle died a few years later, a victim of his cigarettes, and was mourned by a couple of generations of academic physicians whom he had generously supported and mentored. His department had seeded university clinical departments throughout the country with academic leaders. He was not mourned by Mabs MacIntyre. When I had dinner with the MacIntyres in San Francisco shortly after Austin died, she said, 'I hear that that dreadful man Doyle is dead – thank God'. It all depends on your perspective. To me, Austin Doyle was a gifted and generous character. No one is perfect.

During my time at the Repat, I was appointed to the committee for examinations and a little later the board of censors of the Royal Australasian College of Physicians. These were prestigious positions and I was one of the youngest physicians ever to be appointed to them. It started a long and rewarding association with the college. It was a source of considerable collegiality and wonderful for continuing professional education. It also showed that my move from the Royal Melbourne had not led to me slipping totally into obscurity.

I also became active in the Endocrine Society of Australia, a group dedicated to advancing research in the field and was elected to the council and then to the positions of secretary, vice-president and president. I was also appointed to the local organising committee for the International Congress of Endocrinology, the major international conference in the field held only every four years and being staged in Melbourne, the first time in Australia, in 1980. The choice of Melbourne recognised the contribution of a number of Australian researchers to the field and it was a tribute to the international reputation of the chair of the local organising committee, the formidable Bryan Hudson, the foundation professor of medicine at Monash University. The congress was a great success and enhanced the international academic reputation of Melbourne and Australia.

My research was recognised by the award of the Eric Susman Prize by the Royal Australasian College of Physicians, more a recognition of contributions in a number of fields covering insulin release in NZO mice, the role of prostaglandins in the complications of diabetes, the regulation of vitamin D metabolism, the metabolic effects of diphenylhydantoin and the role of intracellular calcium in the effects of caffeine than to a single landmark discovery. As is usually the case, particularly for clinician scientists, I owed much debt to others for this award, particularly at that stage to Jack Martin and to my students and laboratory scientists, including

Marjorie Dunlop, John Wark, Susie Rogers, Lily Stojanovska and Tom Heaney.

One of the tasks we embarked on was to try to develop a specific immunoassay for the active fragment of human parathyroid hormone, the structure of which had been worked out by the Australian Hugh Niall and synthesised by his colleague and fellow Australian Geoff Tregear in the laboratory of John Potts in Boston, as described in an earlier chapter. This necessitated raising antibodies, and goats had been found useful for this. So we immunised some goats and kept them on the farm of a friend of one of our scientists. All went well until the time came to harvest the antibodies. The goats had become accustomed to their life in a free-range environment on the farm. It took much running up hill and down dale and the clever design of funnel-shaped portable fences by our laboratory director, Valdo Michelangeli, and much cheering before we were able to catch the poor goats. We produced – or (to give credit where it is due) the goats produced – antibodies, but they were not as good as the antibodies that became available commercially a little later.

My time at the Repat was critical to the development of my career. It allowed me to have more hands-on involvement in the laboratory and to develop a range of knowledge and experience that I could not have done had I stayed at the Royal Melbourne Hospital.

In 1983 I was appointed as a reader at the University of Melbourne. This quaint title is bestowed in recognition of research achievements and I valued it greatly.

Chapter 7

SAUDI ARABIA, 1981

In 1981 I was invited by the Royal Australasian College of Physicians to spend four weeks in Saudi Arabia teaching endocrinology to the young graduate doctors. This scheme had been an initiative of Peter Little, a fellow of the college who was working in the military hospital in Riyadh. The scheme was that the college would select physicians to spend time at the hospital doing clinical work and teaching the Saudi graduates. The most promising of these young graduates would then be offered registrar positions in Australia to extend their training.

Saudi Arabia at that time was opening up somewhat to the West, but it remained a strict Muslim state ruled by the royal family of the House of Saud, descendants of the legendary Abdul Aziz, who had forcibly united Saudi Arabia earlier in the century.

Society was very conservative. Alcohol was strictly forbidden, although bootlegged Western liquor and home brews of various types ensured that this prohibition was not completely effective. Public beheadings in the city square were still practised. Single women were not allowed to appear in public alone or in the company of a man who was not their husband and were always required to be completely covered by niqab or burqa. The Arab men wore traditional dress. There were no restrictions of mobility and dress for visiting men and I took the opportunity on many occasions to wander downtown to the Gold Souk or Carpet Souk or to eat at little restaurants serving modest but delicious local food.

It was a fascinating time. The hospital was well equipped and many of its staff had trained overseas. It was going through a process of 'localisation', meaning that the largely expatriate specialist staff was gradually being replaced by Saudi nationals. The quality of training of the latter was variable.

The recent graduates comprised a majority who had completed their medical course in Saudi Arabia and one or two who had had their medical education in Pakistan or Egypt. The level of knowledge of those who had trained in Saudi was abysmal and a lot of my time was spent on general medical clinical education at an undergraduate level. The exception was the Pakistani graduate, who was outstanding in every respect. I gave the trainees a multiple choice test at one stage. The Pakistani graduate achieved 120 out of 150, one local graduate 70, and the rest hovered around 10 out of 150. There were negative marks for wrong answers, so this was barely better than guessing.

The Pakistani graduate was brought to Australia as part of the program and did well. He was in love with a Palestinian woman who was training as a radiologist. Despite both being Muslim, they were not allowed to marry in Saudi Arabia because of their different backgrounds. She came to Sydney too and they married secretly. I saw them back in Saudi Arabia when I returned some years later and was pleased that there had not been negative repercussions. The best of the local candidates also came to Australia but did not manage to pass the Australian examinations.

Many of the graduates I was teaching were women. They were relaxed in the hospital and took off their veils. They were very pleasant to teach, but most did not take their studies very seriously. They knew that once they were married, they would not be allowed to work.

The profile of disease in the country was of great interest. Genetic diseases were common because of the traditional practice of consanguineous marriage. Vitamin D deficiency in the women was also common despite the abundant sunshine. The combination of a life spent largely indoors and the almost-complete body covering prevented sunlight exposure, essential to the manufacture of vitamin D by the skin. Rickets was quite common in the babies because of low vitamin D levels in the mothers' breast milk.

The desert-dwelling Bedouins tended to present with advanced disease and many conditions now rare in the West were still prevalent, including rheumatic heart disease and certain specific infections such as schistosomiasis. Added to this, the well-to-do Arabs living in the cities had a high prevalence of lifestyle-related diseases, such as type 2 diabetes, which was present in epidemic proportions, and coronary heart disease. Smoking-related lung disease was also prevalent, owing to the high frequency of smoking.

The appearance of freedom at the hospital was a bit of an illusion. A British doctor who had been working at the Central Hospital for twenty years

CHAPTER 7

remarked to a fellow expatriate doctor after a frustrating gastroenterology outpatient clinic with many of the patients complaining of constipation, 'These people take their bowels even more seriously than their religion'. He was overheard by an interpreter, who reported him to an imam. He was arrested and told he had to pack up and leave the country in twenty-four hours.

A particular drama during my time in Saudi revolved around an old princess, a maiden aunt of the five brothers who have successively ruled Saudi Arabia over the last several decades. Although women are allowed no independent public roles, they are hugely respected within their families. The princess was revered by the Saudi royal family. She was eighty-five and had diabetes. Some weeks before my arrival, she had a stroke. She was in a coma in the royal wing of the military hospital. It was clear that she was not doing well. The medical superintendent of the hospital, an Englishman, was becoming concerned at the level of interest being shown in her health by various high-level dignitaries, including the king and the princes. He arranged for the queen's neurologist and the president of the Royal College of Physicians of London to be flown out from London in the royal family's private jet so they could give their opinion and remove any potential for blame from the hospital staff if her condition deteriorated further.

The distinguished doctors arrived. I escorted them to the princess. They looked at her from the end of the bed and wrote a carefully worded report, which stated that she had had a severe stroke and would not recover. They praised the outstanding medical and nursing care of the hospital staff, which they said was the only reason she had survived to date but that it was inevitable that she would die. A manila envelope changed hands and they departed for the airport. Everyone was most relieved.

It was still thought appropriate that there should be a senior member of staff sleeping in a room in the royal wing in case any misadventure occurred. I was included in the roster for this task. The corridors were filled with various royal attendants and minders of various sorts, who camped there out of respect and solicitude for the princess. It was my turn to sleep in the wing on the night of the visit from the English physicians. I was awoken at midnight and told that Crown Prince Fahd was visiting the princess and wanted to discuss with me what the doctors had said. I stupidly said hello to him in Arabic, but he quickly realised that this was the extent of my knowledge of the language and reverted to perfect English. I explained the poor prognosis and he was satisfied.

The next time it was my turn to sleep in the wing there was more drama. Despite the poor prognosis, it was felt sensible to continue to follow the progress of the princess with a heart monitor. This was displayed on an oscilloscope, where the electrical activity of the heart was shown. She was fading and a sign of this was that she had a period of Cheyne-Stokes respiration – this means that the breathing becomes irregular with periods of twenty or thirty seconds without breathing. All her attendants became anxious and started to gather around from the corridors, despite my trying to calm them down. Amongst much noise and agitation, they started to spin the bed around. They realised that death was imminent and wanted the princess to be pointing towards Mecca. There was much debate about which was the correct direction.

During this commotion, the electrocardiography leads became disconnected. The flat line on the monitor set off great wailing and the prearranged telephone signals to announce that the princess had died was activated. Members of the royal family came from everywhere, but by this time the princess had started to breathe again. I had to explain that she was still alive but very ill. Everyone calmed down, a compass determined the correct direction to Mecca and when the princess finally died the next night when I was not there, everything went more smoothly.

Riyadh was a most interesting city with several beautiful and historic buildings and interesting museums. The desert around was awe-inspiring, with a dramatic escarpment laden with fossils. It had previously been a large inland sea.

I later had two further short visits to Saudi Arabia for seminars. One was devoted to type 2 diabetes, which had become a serious national health problem. As I looked out to my audience of fat men in their white robes, with their large black chauffeur-driven cars waiting outside, I realised that my message that this was a lifestyle-related disease amenable to weight reduction and exercise was falling on deaf ears.

It was sad at these later visits in the 1990s to see that Saudi Arabia was becoming still more conservative once more.

Chapter 8

THE JAMES STEWART CHAIR OF MEDICINE, UNIVERSITY OF MELBOURNE, AT THE ROYAL MELBOURNE HOSPITAL

Dick Lovell had occupied the James Stewart Chair of Medicine at the Royal Melbourne Hospital since it had been founded in 1956. He was due to retire from this position in 1983 after a distinguished period of twenty-eight years. From a room on the foyer of the hospital and a total staff of four or five, the department had grown to occupy two floors of the Clinical Sciences building, which had been constructed in the 1960s. There were about one hundred staff and an active research program in epidemiology, nephrology, arthritis and endocrinology along with other areas. The department was responsible for two general medical units, and in addition, some of the staff had roles in specialist units, notably Priscilla Kincaid-Smith, who was in charge of nephrology, and Ken Muirden, who was in charge of rheumatology. It had become accepted as an important part of the hospital, although the professor of medicine did not have the dominant role in the division of medicine as it had at the Austin Hospital, where the professor was automatically the head of the division.

Although it had not been my single-minded obsession, the position did appeal to me, as it seemed a logical progression from my current role in the department at the Austin and Repatriation hospitals. I had found the combination of clinical work, teaching and research highly rewarding and I felt ready to accept a leadership position in academic medicine. I therefore applied for the position when it was advertised in 1983, with the enthusiastic support of Jack Martin, for which I was very grateful.

NEW TRICKS

Although there were a number of rumours about potential alternative candidates, it turned out that I was the only person interviewed at the final stage. As was the custom at the time, the selection committee was a daunting collection of about twenty-four distinguished university and hospital personnel, chaired by the chancellor of the university, Sir Roy Douglas ('Pansy') Wright. The questioning covered a variety of areas, including the relationship with the Walter and Eliza Hall Institute, the role of the department in the hospital, my vision of the future for the department and the hospital and many other relevant areas. I was a little surprised to be asked by one member of the panel what my view was about banning cigarette advertising, a reflection of a current controversy.

My general principle on such occasions is to say what I thought, which is what I did. I had a phone call from Sir Gustav Nossal, the director of the Walter and Eliza Hall Institute, that evening to say what an interesting interview it had been, which I interpreted as his polite way of saying that I did not have the job. I heard nothing more for two weeks, when I was finally informed that I would be offered the position.

I was forty when I took up the position at the beginning of 1984. Several of the members of the department had been my teachers, including the legendary Priscilla Kincaid-Smith and Bob Fraser. Roger Melick was also the clinical dean responsible for organising the medical student teaching in the hospital. To their credit, they were all very supportive and I gradually grew more comfortable in the role.

I was put through my paces by being asked shortly after I started to conduct a clinicopathological case discussion. This is a form of gladiatorial sport, where a complex case is presented as an unknown to the victim, the so-called expert. The denouement is the revelation of the pathology of the case, which either reveals the clinical mastery of the discussant or is a source of his or her humiliation in the case of a wrong diagnosis.

As I was the professor of medicine, any system was felt to be fair game, rather than only my specialty area of endocrinology. I was presented with a patient who had nodules in the lungs which progressed and ultimately caused the death of the patient. I discussed the case, proposed a diagnosis of nocardiosis, a rare fungal disease, and was proved to be totally wrong. To make it worse, the registrars who were asked their opinion got it right, although I later learnt that they had been acquainted with the case in the hospital. It was a case of a rare vasculitic disease known as lymphomatoid

CHAPTER 8

granulomatosis, a tough one for an endocrinologist, who had, till that stage, never seen a case.

As it happened, it is a favourite for such clinicopathological presentations and on two later occasions at different hospitals I correctly diagnosed it. The staff of the hospital was kind to me after my public display of ignorance.

After the great strides made by Lovell, the department of medicine was now well accepted by the hospital staff and, given that I had trained at the hospital and had been a member of the senior medical staff, the old 'town and gown' divide had well and truly been laid to rest. Nevertheless, the influence of the university in the hospital was still suboptimal, as the university department was responsible for two medical units and its members were not fully integrated into the rest of the clinical services of the hospital, with the exception of nephrology and rheumatology, where a university staff member headed the unit.

My ambition was to achieve a much greater integration of the university and hospital staff, with the academic philosophy of combining clinical care with a commitment to education and advancing knowledge through research permeating the whole hospital. To me, this is the essence of a 'teaching hospital' and it should not be dependent on whether the clinician's salary is being paid by the university, by the hospital or by a combination of the two. The visiting staff, who may have a commitment ranging from 0.1 to 0.6 of their time to the hospital, should also share this philosophy, even if their other commitments do not allow them to play an active role in research.

We attempted to achieve greater integration by reorganising the general medical units so that the academic staff was spread throughout the five general medical units. We also tried to link specialist units with general units so that even subspecialists would share some general medical responsibilities. This was based on the successful model then operating at Flinders Medical Centre in Adelaide under the leadership of John Chalmers. There was some resistance to this from the specialist physicians and this experiment did not work well. However, in contrast to several similar teaching hospitals around the country, the general medical units remained strong. This was helpful in the training of the interns and registrars and also of benefit to many of the patients who presented either with undifferentiated disease or with problems affecting multiple systems. I remain convinced that a well-trained general physician, often with some particular subspecialty interest, is a very necessary and valuable component of the medical workforce, both within and outside the teaching hospital environment. Certainly, it is this form of general internist who is most often sought by general practitioners or by surgeons seeking assessment and oversight of the patients on whom they are operating.

In contrast to the lack of success in integrating the general and specialist units, the sprinkling of academic staff between the various units was successful and did lead to a greater engagement of the university with the hospital. I also took over the role of chairing the division of medicine's weekly lunchtime forum and chairing the division of medicine itself. This was not because I needed those roles, but because I felt it essential that the head of the university's department of medicine should be very visible within the hospital and in a position to have a political influence. This should ensure that the priorities of the hospital are aligned with the requirements of teaching and research, those elements that the academic units within hospitals were there to enhance. My activities in these roles were well accepted and I was never conscious of any anti-academic prejudice among my colleagues – indeed, I enjoyed a most productive and collaborative environment with the doctors, nurses, other staff and the administration.

Another challenge early in my time as professor of medicine was to get a more productive relationship with the clinical research unit of the Walter and Eliza Hall Institute (WEHI), headed by Ian Mackay. Mackay was a notable clinical immunologist who had made substantial contributions to the understanding of autoimmune diseases, especially what was then known as lupoid hepatitis, now more often known as non-viral or autoimmune active chronic hepatitis. Ian ran a clinical unit in the hospital and a research laboratory in the Hall Institute. I considered that his objectives of furthering clinical or translational research and those of the department of medicine overlapped. Moreover, building bridges between the department and the Walter and Eliza Hall Institute seemed to me to be highly desirable. I also wished to bring basic scientists and clinicians closer together. So, I suggested to Ian that we should start a fortnightly series entitled 'Clinical Science Forum', with the responsibility for organising the presentations alternating between the clinical research unit of WEHI and the university's department of medicine. The idea was that each presentation should have a theme centred around a clinical problem, with clinical and basic researchers presenting work directed at resolving the identified issues. It might start with a case presentation or a clinical description working back to the research intended

CHAPTER 8

to resolve the problems, or it might start with a description of a disease and describe basic work then developed into a potential therapeutic or diagnostic approach.

The fora were a success for a period of time, with some outstanding sessions. They served a useful purpose, although after a few years they had run their course with time-poor researchers and clinicians finding it difficult to organise the presentations to sufficient standard and to attend fora where the relevance of the subject matter might not have been immediately apparent.

It is difficult for clinical professors to find time to interact with students so that the professor of a discipline can truly be in a position to influence the education and attitudes of a new generation of students. I had been attracted to academic medicine in part by my love of teaching. I very much enjoyed the bedside tutorials I gave regularly to the small groups of students allocated to my general medical ward and the general medical and endocrine teaching in outpatients. I also gave occasional teaching on endocrinology topics to earlier years of the medical course and during the lecture program in fourth year. But I wished for a more active role and started a problem-based teaching format in general medicine for the final-year students at the hospital. This consisted of the presentation of a case each week to the eighty or so final-year students at the hospital and then asking questions of the students going along the rows. I tried to learn as many names as I could and to make it as much fun as possible. The students all felt sufficiently involved and challenged to be on edge, but I tried to avoid overly embarrassing individual students by passing quickly on if they did not know the answers or throwing it open to the whole class if the question was difficult. The students seemed to enjoy it and I was voted the teacher of the year by the students on three occasions, an honour that I particularly valued.

Research was exciting during this period. Along with the head of my laboratory, Marjorie Dunlop, a recently appointed senior lecturer, Joe Proietto, and a National Health and Medical Research Council (NHMRC) senior research fellow, Kerin O'Dea, we successfully applied for an NHMRC program grant on the causes and complications of diabetes. There were many synergies between the work that Joe did on the role of hepatic glucose production and insulin resistance in the aetiology of type two diabetes, Kerin's work on nutritional influences on diabetes and on diabetes in Indigenous communities and our own work on insulin release and on diabetic complications focusing on the role of prostanoids and aldose reductase. By the time of the renewal of the program grant, Kerin O'Dea had been appointed as professor of human nutrition at Deakin University, and Stella Clark joined the group as one of the chief investigators. Stella's interest in signal transduction complemented some of Marjorie's interests and added an additional dimension to the program.

The program spanned the spectrum, extending from clinical and population research to animal research, tissue culture and molecular medicine, eventually bringing in transgenic technology. Many significant publications and invitations to speak at international meetings and other forms of recognition resulted. As the head of a large university department, with additional roles within the hospital and outside, especially at this time with the Endocrine Society of Australia and the Royal Australasian College of Physicians, it was difficult to make room for hands-on laboratory work. At that time, my contributions were in weekly group discussions and weekly meetings with the postgraduate students I supervised. I played a significant role in writing grant applications and papers, but I cannot emphasise too strongly how dependent I was on my research students, colleagues and particularly Marjorie Dunlop to continue the momentum of our research.

There was little time to interact in the politics of the university outside the hospital. The politics of health and of the hospital, together with clinical, teaching and research activities and involvement with the College of Physicians, the Endocrine Society and NHMRC, was fully engaging and time consuming. Although a member of the professorial board of the university, I was not able to attend as regularly as I would have liked. Graeme Ryan, the very efficient and effective dean of the faculty after David Penington had finished his term, made it clear that my primary responsibility was to get the interactions with the hospital and health service right as well as the usual expectation of delivering the highest quality education and research. He said that he could take care of the interests of the faculty at the university level. It is unfortunately a fact of life that the other calls make it difficult for clinical professors to become fully involved with the university to which they are appointed. It was only later that I realised the richness that comes from a closer involvement with the multitude of disciplines and skills represented in a comprehensive research-intensive university.

Chapter 9

CHINA, 1985

In 1985 I was invited by the Australia-China Project, an aid program administered by the University of Queensland, to spend four weeks teaching the doctors and residents at the affiliated hospital of the Shandong Medical College, later to become the Shandong Medical University, in Jinan, Shandong Province. Jinan is six hours by train from Beijing on the route to Shanghai, which was a further twelve hours away. Shandong at that time was described as an isolated backwater of seventy million people. I am sure it has a much larger population now, and compared with more remote provinces, it was hardly isolated. Nevertheless, till that time it had been largely bypassed by the West. My role was to give a series of lectures and to discuss cases in the wards with the postgraduate medical staff and with all the specialists in endocrinology. I was told to come with about thirteen lectures prepared.

The hospital itself was fairly well equipped and had access to most of the relevant Western drugs. There was a CT scanner, although this mostly lay idle because of lack of technologists to repair it when it malfunctioned.

My visit revealed how essential good education is in preparing doctors to deliver care that is appropriate to the needs of patients. Apart from the old professor who had received his education before the cultural revolution, the other endocrinologists had received their medical education during the cultural revolution from staff who had been recruited from the peasantry, while the educated doctors who represented the 'bourgeoisie' were sent to work in the fields. Hence, they were incredibly ignorant and lacking fundamental clinical skills. Frighteningly, they were responsible for the education of the next generation of doctors, the eager and intelligent young students to whom I had been asked to give a teaching session or two.

The standard of English amongst the staff was also very poor, although it was much better amongst the younger doctors and students. My interpreter was a delightful nephrologist of about sixty years of age, who had learnt his English from his father, who in turn had learnt it from the Germans when they occupied Shandong seventy or so years earlier. Not surprisingly, the quality of the translation left a lot to be desired. This was apparent when I gave my first lecture and made a couple of light-hearted comments, which I had hoped would at least raise a polite ripple of laughter, but instead were greeted with a look of profound puzzlement. Fortunately, my slides were fairly clear and comprehensive and the written English word seemed to be understood better than the spoken word.

The lectures themselves were quite a performance. They usually began with an intricate process of getting the primitive slide projector connected to the equally primitive power point, usually by joining several non-insulated wires in a most precarious fashion. The lectures themselves, including time for translation, would take two hours. There would then be a period of silence, during which, after the first lecture, I prepared to leave. Then the old professor asked a question. This was followed by other questions in a hierarchical sequence, descending from the more senior doctors until another hour had elapsed. After I had completed the thirteen prepared lectures in endocrinology, I was asked to give additional lectures, which I prepared hastily in areas outside my major expertise, such as onco (cancer) genes and gastrointestinal hormones. I prepared these lectures hastily the night before, comfortable that although I was not expert in these areas, I knew considerably more than my audience.

The morning case presentations were even more of a performance. They would typically be attended by forty or so residents and senior doctors. The discussion would start with the presentation of the clinical case by one of the residents and then, with great ceremony, I would be taken to see the case. I would ask a question or two and then examine the patient as appropriate to the case. I was then escorted to a cold tap over a 'gully trap', where I was invited to wash my hands and to dry them on a cold, dirty, wet, grey towel. One of my predecessors from Australia had explained to the hospital staff that it was good practice to wash hands before and after examining patients, but the solution seemed more likely to do harm than good. After the examination of the patient was complete, we would retire to a tutorial room to discuss the case for the rest of the morning. The whole performance was timed to take three hours and if I felt like stopping sooner, the flow of questions would ensure that the full three hours were occupied.

CHAPTER 9

It was during these presentations that the appalling level of clinical care became apparent. Despite there being a huge shortage of beds needed for admission of sick patients, the current patients were kept in hospital for weeks on end, with little being done for them. Diagnoses were frequently wrong and treatment almost invariably suboptimal. My task was to be both diplomatic and instructive. It was important that I should not humiliate the doctors in charge of the case by pointing out elementary errors in management. On the other hand, if we did not work through to the correct diagnosis and treatment, my visit would be wasted.

One week of cases was particularly frustrating, as in that week, every case presented to me was obviously misdiagnosed with elementary mistakes in interpretation. For example, I was presented with a case described as Addison's disease (failure of the adrenal glands associated with tiredness, low blood pressure and skin pigmentation along with characteristically low plasma cortisol level without the normal fluctuation from morning to night). The case seemed strange from the beginning, as the cortisol levels were not low and showed normal diurnal fluctuation and the blood pressure was not low. When questioned, the normal cortisols were ascribed to laboratory error. We saw the patient, who clearly had darker skin than most Han Chinese. I asked him about whether others in his village had skin pigmentation and he said that it was common. Apparently, there had been considerable genetic mixing with a dark-skinned minority group generations before. Other cases that week included a patient with fibrous dysplasia of bone misdiagnosed as hyperparathyroid bone disease despite normal calcium levels and a young man with hypertension secondary to renal disease misdiagnosed as a tumour of the adrenal gland producing adrenaline because of falsely elevated reading for adrenaline products in the urine, really due to a well-known effect of one of the drugs being used to treat his high blood pressure. And so it went on. Each time I was presented with such misdiagnosis, my heart would sink and I would think of a strategy to work through to the correct diagnosis without the professor losing face. I must have succeeded to his satisfaction, as on my departure, he presented me with two bottles of maotai, the foul tasting and foul smelling, highly alcoholic Chinese spirit. Or maybe it was punishment.

At that time, Chinese clinicians were claiming outstanding clinical success with human foetal pancreatic islet transplantation to reverse insulin-dependent diabetes. Much work had been done on this in the

Western world with a notable lack of success. I was very interested to find out more. Initially, when I asked for details and results, the doctors were evasive. But the topic arose again following one of the case presentations. It was an eighteen-year-old girl with insulin-dependent diabetes, which she had had since the age of twelve or so. She had been treated with once-daily long-acting insulin. She had features of what is known as Mauriac's syndrome – this has virtually disappeared in the Western world, as it develops as the result of extremely poorly controlled diabetes. It is characterised by poor growth, low body weight, delayed puberty and an enlarged liver due to fatty infiltration. This girl had all these features and was described as a case of failed insulin treatment. I was told that she was going to be treated with foetal pancreatic islet transplantation. Modern treatment with multiple insulin injections per day or an insulin infusion pump would have been much more effective.

When I later respectfully asked once more for information on the experience of the team with foetal pancreatic islet transplantation, this was provided. The islets were obtained from up to eight foetuses at a time. The foetuses were of up to eight months of gestation. The condition of the patients was 'improved' by transplantation. It is clear that at that time, practices were condoned in China (at least in this provincial centre) that would never be contemplated in Australia and which no ethics committee would approve if they were.

There were substantial efforts to merge traditional Chinese medicine with Western medicine. The prevailing philosophy was that the two forms of medicine would benefit from each other. It was clear to me, however, that the underlying philosophies are so far apart that the two approaches are incompatible. Western medicine attempts precise diagnosis in terms of aetiology and pathology relating to a particular organ or body system. Chinese medicine is directed towards body regions and symptoms. It does not depend, as does Western medicine, on a scientific theoretical underpinning based on biochemistry, physiology, anatomy, microbiology and pathology. Although some Western doctors have chosen to incorporate components of Chinese medicine into their practice, it is not founded on scientific compatibility of the approaches.

The Affiliated University Hospital was essentially based around Western medicine, although it did have a traditional Chinese component as well. I asked if I could visit the traditional Chinese medicine hospital nearby and

CHAPTER 9

this was arranged towards the end of my visit. I was very impressed by the diabetes patients who seemed significantly fitter than those I had seen in the Western hospital. I asked how they were treated. I was told by acupuncture, various extracts of this and that, and then to my surprise, insulin. Respectfully, I asked why insulin was also used – didn't the traditional treatments work? I was told that they did, but they took some time to be effective, so insulin was used in the meantime!

The pharmacy of the traditional hospital was particularly impressive. From a control panel that one might expect to see in the cockpit of a jet airliner, the pharmacist pushed an array of buttons. These activated levers, which opened the lids of inverted tin cans that looked like old-style biscuit containers. This process dispensed contents ranging from plants to animal, fish and shell extracts on to a plate, which was transported from tin to tin on a conveyer belt. At the end of this process, the assembled ingredients were boiled up together to form a 'concoction' to be administered to the patient.

There was a huge enthusiasm by all the young students to learn English. About 10 per cent of the brightest students were selected at the beginning of the course to study medicine in English. They spent their first year learning English before proceeding to the rest of the course. For the first two weeks of my time in Jinan, I was accompanied by Caroline. Each lunchtime, in the two-hour break for lunch and a 'rest', we would get a knock on the door, and two Chinese students would come and say that they had come to practise their English. We had some delightful conversations and learnt a lot about the lives of these young Chinese.

One lunchtime, an earnest young man announced that he was the president of the local English club and he would like to invite Caroline to deliver a talk to the club about Australia. She asked how many people might come and she was told about forty and accepted. She had had the foresight to get some slides from the Victorian Tourist Bureau.

My experience at giving lectures had suggested to me that this could be quite a performance and I was not disappointed. For a start, the president had underestimated the size of the audience. The whole floor above the library had been chosen as a venue – a huge space. People were crowded to occupy all the space and bulged out the doors – there must have been 600 people. There was the usual delay as our hosts tried to rig up the projector with Heath Robinson joins between bare wires and power points. Eventually all was in readiness, although the length of the lead meant that the projected image was far too small for the vast hall.

Caroline performed admirably. A notable feature was that every time she pointed out some animal or object on the slides, there was an echo from 600 voices as they pronounced the words.

At the end of Caroline's talk, she invited questions. There was the customary silence for a while until eventually a hand went up and one of the students delicately asked, 'Is it true that in Australia, boys and girls can go out together before they are married?'

To a general quiet giggle, Caroline replied that yes, this did happen.

Another pause, then another question from someone else, 'And is it true that boys and girls sometimes hold hands before they are married?'

Caroline answered yes to greater mirth.

Next, another question. 'And is it true that they sometimes kiss each other before they are married?'

Caroline answered yes and decided that it was an appropriate point to end the question time!

We were extremely kindly treated by our hosts and had a couple of weekends sightseeing around Beijing, including all the usual sights, such as the Great Wall, Ming Tombs, Forbidden City, Tiananmen Square, the Temple of Heaven and the Summer Palace. We also had a couple of days sightseeing in Shandong, including visiting Confucius' birthplace in Qufu and climbing Tai Shan (Holy Mountain). It is said that if you climb Tai Shan, you will be healthy for the next year. Given the strenuous nature of the climb, I was cynical enough to consider it a good stress test rather than a reflection of the holy powers of the mountain. There were many old ladies, some with bound feet, making the climb to ensure their survival for another year. We were escorted down by young students, exhorting us to be careful and taking the opportunity to practise their English.

We also took the opportunity to visit a village medical centre. This was run by a Chinese traditional doctor and the usual impressive array of plant and animal products with miraculous powers of healing and enhancement were on display. Impressively, he was able to produce the health records, including immunisation records of all the members of his village. The organised nature of Chinese society has allowed very effective implementation of public health programs. This has led to a substantial increase in life expectancy, despite the shortcomings in one-on-one treatment of illness.

CHAPTER 9

There was a disappointing postscript to the China visit and the Australia-China project. At the end of my visit, I was asked to nominate one of the local endocrinologists to come to Australia for a year to work and study with me at the Royal Melbourne Hospital. I thought that the mid-level endocrinologists were not likely to benefit much – their basic knowledge and English skills were not at a level where they could fully engage with the opportunities in Australia. On the other hand, there were some recent graduates with excellent English, eager to learn and with sufficient basic medical knowledge to benefit enormously. I recommended one of these. Perhaps not surprisingly, politics won, and a forty-year-old endocrinologist was chosen. Dr Wang was a delightful man. He came equipped with an embossed tea set as a gift for us, which he had carried on his lap all the way from Jinan. He had left his wife and young child behind in Jinan. Unfortunately, despite his efforts and ours, I fear that he derived little benefit from his visit.

I have returned to China on a number of occasions since that first visit. The progress in all aspects of medicine as well as other areas of science has been quite remarkable, as I will outline in a later chapter.

Chapter 10

CASEMIX FUNDING AND THE 'CRISIS' IN THE HOSPITALS IN THE 1990s

Money has always been tight in large hospitals around the world. Where care is funded by taxes, demand will always be high and greater than the will of governments to pay for it. So, tough financial times are a fact of life in our hospital system. This leads to the need to prioritise care so that the sickest have access. To the credit of administrators and health care professionals in Australia, it is still fair to say that for really sick patients, the care in our teaching hospitals is at least as good as that provided to the general public anywhere in the world.

The combination of providing such good care to really sick patients and working with constrained budgets means that there are often long queues for elective patients awaiting surgery for less urgent but often very painful conditions, such as joint replacement for arthritis or coronary artery surgery in situations that are apparently not life-threatening. It also means that emergency departments are not staffed to cope with peak periods of demand and bed numbers are insufficient to cope with need. A difficult equilibrium can be achieved, but this is fragile and the ability of opposition political parties to use waiting lists, trolleys waiting in emergency departments and ambulance bypass of emergency departments for political advantage means that there is a lot of knee jerk decision making that distorts sound management and planning. Money is not the only answer, as the difficulties created by the division between commonwealth and state responsibilities for health care also contribute substantially.

In the 1980s, times were becoming more difficult in the hospital system as a series of financial bungles and external financial difficulties afflicted the dying days of the Cain and Kirner Labor governments. But despite thinking

CHAPTER 10

at that time how difficult things were for our hospitals, they were relatively spared compared with what came later.

When the Kennett Liberal and National Party government came to power in 1992, Victoria was in a financial mess and the feisty combination of Kennett and his treasurer, Alan Stockdale, set about what they regarded as setting things right. Given the significant budget demands of the public hospitals, it is not surprising that they were a target and their budgets were significantly cut. This was soon compounded by the introduction of 'casemix' funding. Up until then, the budgets for hospitals had to a large extent been historically determined, with broad agreements negotiated between the state government and the hospitals about the budget they would work towards. There were variations if the hospital was to take on an extra load through amalgamations or other perturbations, or there might be global cuts in times of financial stringency. So-called 'teaching hospitals' received more funds than their load of patients would appear to justify to take into account their teaching, postgraduate training and research roles and because of a greater degree of complexity of their case load. But this was done largely in an ad hoc manner.

In association with other measures designed to improve economic management in the state, casemix funding was introduced. Essentially, this is a complex system of attributing a certain number of bed days to designated conditions, with allowances for complicating factors. This determines the funding to be allocated for that condition. If the patient is kept in hospital longer, the hospital carried the cost. If the patient is discharged earlier, it is to the advantage of the hospital's budget. Thus, there are incentives for the people in the hospital responsible for the budget to encourage earlier discharge.

These signals are appropriate if they are not to the detriment of the patient's care. Unfortunately, the budget incentive tended to encourage inappropriately early discharge, with patients unable to care for themselves, more demands on health care in the general community and great difficulties for families and carers. Many examples of patients requiring early readmission to cope with complications arising from early discharge were seen.

There are other problems with this system. The precise sequence of recording the primary illness or procedure and the listing of complicating factors can have a substantial effect on the funding attracted by the case. This led to a growing industry of maximising income through adjusting the nature of the recorded cause for admission and 'game playing'. Admissions were recorded for patients in the emergency department and because outpatient treatment did not attract casemix funding, there was an incentive to admit patients rather than to treat them as outpatients, at least until another scheme was thought up.

There was one component of the new scheme which had a profound beneficial effect, at least for a time. This was a throughput bonus pool. This meant that if the hospital treated more than the negotiated number of cases adjusted for casemix, it would be paid for the extra cases treated. For the first time, there was a financial incentive for the hospital to become more efficient and to reduce its waiting lists. There was a perceptible difference in the mood in the hospitals. Everyone worked harder, knowing that not only would this have the desired effect of reducing waiting lists and relieving pain and misery, it would not be a financial cost for the hospital to do so. Unfortunately, this scheme was short-lived. The government found that it was costing too much, even though each patient treated was at the agreed cost. So the throughput pool was soon capped at levels well below that needed to meet demand. This, of course, led to waiting lists blowing out again, trolleys in the emergency departments, ambulance bypass and political vulnerability for the government.

The department of health reacted in a typical way to the political pressure now caused by all the measured parameters deteriorating. It devised financial penalties for hospitals if waiting lists exceeded certain levels, if waiting times in emergency were exceeded, or emergency departments were put on standby more often than specified. In other words, although the hospitals were funded only to treat a certain number of cases well below the demand, if the indicators that demand was not being met rose, they would be financially penalised. They could not afford to treat the number of patients that would have to be treated to avoid penalties, and they could not afford the penalties. It was a catch-22 situation that, to mix my literary satirical allusions, would have made Sir Humphrey of *Yes, Minister* proud.

Not surprisingly, the hospitals started to devise ways around the penalties – not so much in their own interests, but to allow them to function adequately and to try to meet demand. Patients awaiting admission were not put on waiting lists, but on alternative lists indicating that they would be added to the waiting lists later. Parts of the emergency departments were declared to be wards, so that waiting times in the department would seem to have decreased. This was intensely frustrating to hospital staff, and morale, which had risen with the throughput bonus, plummeted.

CHAPTER 10

It was in this environment that I attended the wind-up meeting for 1993 of the Clinical Casemix Advisory Committee, of which I was a member. The late Marie Tehan, a well-meaning minister for health out of her depth in the shark-infested waters of the portfolio at a time of government cost constraints, came into the meeting and said that we should all congratulate ourselves on the successful introduction of casemix funding. This was the final straw for me. I said that up until the time of the capping of the throughput bonus pool there had been positive effects, but since then, with funding set far below demand and penalties imposed for failing to meet demand, the hospitals had been placed in an impossible position and the system was falling apart. Not surprisingly, this was not well received by the minister, who may well not have been aware of what was really going on in the hospitals.

Shortly after, the professors of medicine at each of the major teaching hospitals affiliated with the University of Melbourne, Colin Johnston from the Austin, Jack Martin from St Vincent's and I decided to write a letter to the *Age* newspaper indicating our despair at the funding cuts and the impact on quality of care and on teaching and research. We tried to make the letter apolitical, emphasising the particular role that the teaching hospitals played in the education and postgraduate training of the doctors and nurses of the future and in safeguarding quality of care throughout the health system. We stated that it was not possible to evaluate the benefits or otherwise of the casemix system of funding when it was accompanied by such savage funding cuts that the quality of care was threatened independent of the funding mechanism.

Second-hand reports suggested that the minister subsequently phoned the university's vice-chancellor, David Penington, to ask him why he had allowed his professors to write a letter like this. According to the reports the vice-chancellor replied that he had not known of our intention (which was true), but if he had known, he would not have tried to stop us, and if he had tried to stop us, we would not have taken any notice. The second and third parts of this response, if accurately reported, were hypothetical, as they were not tested.

There were other elements of the new government's introduction of the new funding system combined with funding cuts. One was that the casemix system, if implemented in a pure form, would have had a devastating effect on teaching hospitals. This was recognised by the architect of the scheme, the noted health economist Stephen Duckett, on the Friday before the week in which the scheme was due to be announced. Stephen assembled three people, including me, to give advice on how the extra costs of postgraduate training of health professionals should be taken into account. A whiteboard was produced and the costs and slow-down impacts of having doctors in training ranging from interns through to registrars were estimated and these were factored into the formulae. It was a rough-and-ready bidding system, with no science or evidence base, but it played a vital role in ensuring that there was at least some prospect of the major teaching hospitals surviving under this system. Of course, the extra weightings were not merely associated with the training function. They were also a reflection of the increased complexity of the cases seen in the tertiary hospitals, which was not adequately dealt with by the weights assigned in the casemix system, but to admit this would have been to recognise a basic flaw in the system.

Another element dealt with in a pragmatic and fundamentally illegal way was the cost of delivering care in the outpatient departments of the major hospitals. The outpatient department was an important component of the hospitals, as it allowed patients with complex illness to receive continuity of care from the doctors of the unit which had cared for them in the hospital. It was also the venue for providing specialist opinion for patients referred from general practitioners in the community, who could be better investigated and treated in the environment of a teaching hospital or who could not afford additional costs incurred in the private sector. Outpatient clinics provided an excellent teaching environment, with patients often presenting with undifferentiated and undiagnosed problems or ongoing symptoms and signs not often seen in the frenetic environment of inpatient wards.

The problem was that the funds provided by the commonwealth government for the hospitals were perceived by the hospital administrators and by the state government bureaucrats to be insufficient to fund adequately these services. We were thus specifically instructed by the department of health officials and by the hospital administrators to bulk-bill these services to Medicare. This would effectively transfer costs from the hospital and the state government to the commonwealth government. This was in contravention of the Australian Health Care Agreement. We were also told to write outside prescriptions for Pharmaceutical Benefits Scheme medications for patients being discharged and for patients in outpatients instead of prescribing the medication from the hospital pharmacy. This also transferred costs from the

CHAPTER 10

hospital to the commonwealth. It was an immensely frustrating time, as neither of these subterfuges saved the taxpayer money, but merely transferred costs from the state to the commonwealth. But because the hospitals were so poorly funded, we had to comply to allow us to come close to providing reasonable care for the patients who needed it.

About this time, Jenny Macklin, later to become a federal minister, was asked to prepare a national health strategy for the commonwealth government. This came out as a series of position papers which identified the complexity of the 'jigsaw' relating to the number and variety of agencies responsible for delivering health and aged care at the state and commonwealth levels. These papers followed extensive consultations and correctly identified the many inefficiencies and dysfunctionalities in the system and suggested ways to resolve these. These included models for integrated care and better prevention and community care to alleviate pressure on the acute care hospitals. Along with the prevailing philosophy at the time, the Macklin strategy foresaw decreased requirement for hospital beds in the future, as average length of stay for each admission was decreasing and more surgery was being done as day procedures. Moreover, it was hoped that better preventive strategies and community-based care would decrease the need for hospital admissions.

I took issue with this when I met with Jenny Macklin and she asked me to prepare a paper articulating my views and their rationale. I did this, pointing out that there were finite limits to the reduction in length of stay, that the ageing of the population would lead to increased, not decreased, demand for all health services, including hospital inpatient beds for joint replacements, coronary artery surgery and strokes, amongst other problems, and that there were also unpredictable demands that would come from new and re-emergent diseases such as HIV-AIDS. I received no response to this paper and the strategy continued to propagate the myth of decreasing requirements for hospital beds into the future. All our states are experiencing the consequences of this misjudgement at present.

A similar lack of alignment between aspiration and reality was seen in the forward planning for mental health services. Victoria, along with other states, was recognising that the old-style asylums of the past were not an appropriate or humane way to deal with chronic mental illness, such as schizophrenia. Moreover, modern drugs allowed many such patients to be treated safely in the community. The extrapolation that all such specialised mental hospitals could be closed and all the patients returned to the community was not justified by evidence, and attempts to achieve this continue to have undesirable consequences. The large amount of funding required to provide adequate supervised community housing for the significant number of chronically ill patients unable to fend for themselves was not made available; instead, patients were discharged to community settings with inadequate support. Drug and alcohol abuse, homelessness and sometimes suicide or crime resulted. Although there is no wish to return to the past, both short and long-term specialised hospital care and accommodation for patients with mental illness are urgently needed for the significant minority of patients who cannot fend for themselves in the community and who cannot be adequately looked after in that environment.

At the time of the drive by the Kennett government to increase the efficiencies of the public hospitals, a move was made to increase the management efficiency by bringing into hospitals senior administrators who had a proven record of management in private industry or government departments but who had no content knowledge of health care. The philosophy was that management principles needed to be applied to make the hospitals efficient, and these principles were not dependent on what product was to be delivered. The governing boards of the hospitals were also reformulated to remove, to a large extent, specific health care expertise and to replace this expertise with more financial and legal skills. While it is true that such skills are required and most of the new boards were composed of well-meaning and capable people, it did lead to a dangerous dependence on the input from the CEO and a lack of a clear comprehension by the boards of the diverse range of functions that a public hospital had to fulfil. Financial and legal aspects became the focus for the boards, with less than appropriate attention to the quality of care, the role of the hospital in teaching and research and the extent to which the needs of the community were being met.

The discontent of the medical and nursing staff of the hospitals about the consequences of the budget constraints, the change in the funding model and the changes in governance and management became a major political crisis in the mid 1990s. The premier, Jeff Kennett, responded by cancelling his Christmas vacation one year, stating that he was going to visit the teaching hospitals personally to assess the so-called 'crisis' in the hospitals. When he visited the Royal Melbourne Hospital, he said that it had been put to him that the dual commonwealth-state funding for health care was

CHAPTER 10

a cause of dysfunctionality and that it would be best if the state handed the responsibility of all health care funding, including hospital funding, over to the commonwealth. What did we think of that? We agreed that the division was a cause for dysfunctionality and having only one government, such as the commonwealth, responsible for health funding and care was a good idea. The premier seemed to nod in agreement.

Some months later, Mr Kennett reported on the outcome of his tour of the hospitals. He correctly reported that he had suggested that the state could hand responsibility for funding and running the hospitals to the commonwealth, but said that he had been persuaded by the hospital staff that they did not wish that! This was certainly not the message we gave him at the Royal Melbourne Hospital, but of course, we could not comment on what he had heard elsewhere.

Given that it represents one of the major areas of state responsibility, it is unlikely that any state would willingly give up their role in running hospitals. Why would not schools, roads, public transport and police follow, leaving nothing substantial for the states?

Many of us look back nostalgically to the time when hospitals were, to a large extent, run by altruistic doctors and nurses, with patients able to receive the best of care then available and students had access to plenty of patients able to give good histories and to enjoy and benefit from the students' interest. The relationship between doctors and nurses was hierarchical and paternalistic, but there was, by and large, mutual respect and a highly collaborative atmosphere.

It was inevitable, however, with the evolution of sophisticated and expensive technology and the demands placed on the system by growth in number and the ageing of the population, that the old way could not continue. The predominantly female nursing staff correctly rebelled against its 'handmaiden' status, and the old patriarchal model was changed forever. Bed stays shortened and the admitted patients were sicker, so students had less access to patients. More emphasis was put on financial performance and on easily measured political pressure points, such as waiting lists, ambulance bypass of emergency departments and waiting time for patients on trolleys in the emergency department. Interns and residents had regulated hours and the number of beds per nurse was strictly regulated.

Many of the changes have been for the better and others are the inevitable consequences of stresses on the system from the increased capacity to deliver high technology care and the costs of such care. It does not stop the nostalgia for what has been lost!

The Rudd-Gillard government 'health reforms' included the intention of sharing the direct funding of hospitals with the states and the introduction of an activity-based funding formula across the country with governance of the hospitals through networks with their own boards – virtually the system already operating in Victoria. So despite its shortcomings, the Victorian system has been taken as an exemplar for the rest of the country. The commonwealth government has now changed and it is not clear how the system of commonwealth-state funding of health care will evolve.

In any new scheme, allowance should be made for teaching and research roles of large hospitals and diseconomies of scale in small rural hospitals. The new proposals do not adequately address the key issue of continuity of care between hospitals and the community. Moreover, a private system largely subsidised on an uncapped fee-for-service basis is not financially sustainable in the long term, despite its popularity with the public and the political cost of changing it. As the shortage of doctors is overcome, the design of the system will make it become more and more expensive.

The emphasis of Medicare on rewarding acute episodes of care for intermittent disease is also poorly suited to the health needs of the community. With the changing demographics and pattern of disease, more emphasis on maintenance of health in those with chronic diseases and in disease prevention is required.

An extension of the current proposal could see divisions of general practice or their successors, medicare locals, included in the networks. The universities with medical schools have developed very effective relationships with their teaching hospitals, regional hospitals and divisions of general practice, and David Penington has suggested that these partnerships could serve as the basis for local health networks responsible not only for patient care, but also for health promotion and disease prevention, for health professional education and for translational research. Funding could be on a per-capita basis, adjusted for age profile and socio-economic status of the regions being served. Only through such a system, where the same body is responsible for prevention and treatment and care in the hospital and community, will there be a more rational and optimal use of the available resources with maximum benefit to the community.

CHAPTER 10

With better coordination of care across the various parts of the health system, a changed remuneration system, a more rational approach to use of 'futile' treatments, particularly towards the end of life, and less defensive investigations to guard against the risk of medical negligence claims, there is the potential for considerable improvement in the quality of care and the outcomes for patients without extra cost. Currently, our political system, our administrative structures and our insurance and legal systems make it very unlikely that the required changes will occur any time soon.

Chapter 11

MEDICAL EDUCATION, THE MEDICAL WORKFORCE AND THE DOHERTY COMMITTEE OF INQUIRY

The perceived knowledge and communication skills of doctors are always political issues, given the central role that health and health care play in communities around the world. In addition, the costs of health care in developed countries and the role that the medical workforce plays in generating these costs causes anxiety about the medical workforce. The increasing costs of the government-funded Medicare system in Australia in the 1980s led to a particular concern that an oversupply of doctors might be generating excessive costs. The dual concerns about medical education on the one hand and the size of the medical workforce led the Hawke-Keating government to set up the Committee of Inquiry into Medical Education and the Workforce in 1987 to report to both the minister of health, Neal Blewett and the minister of education, John Dawkins. The committee was to be chaired by Ralph Doherty, a noted medical academic and researcher who was the pro vice-chancellor of health sciences at the University of Queensland, having previously been the dean of medicine at the university.

I was invited to be a member of the seven-person committee and readily accepted. This was an important process and I felt that it was essential that someone directly involved in traditional medical education, aware of both the strengths and weaknesses of the process, should be involved. Other members of the committee were Delys Sargent, a social scientist who had worked at the University of Melbourne, Neville Hicks, a historian from the University of Adelaide, Sue Morey, a public health doctor and senior medical bureaucrat in the New South Wales department of health, Bernard Amos,

CHAPTER 11

the CEO of Westmead Hospital in Sydney and Robert Smith, a geographer who was vice-chancellor of the University of Western Australia. There was substantial secretarial and project support from the commonwealth department of health. The inquiry was launched with great fanfare and there was significant interest in the inquiry from medical schools, the Australian Medical Association and other medical bodies, the newly formed Australian Medical Council, and a wide variety of consumer groups.

As in all such processes where a disparate group is brought together, it is always a little uncertain how the committee will function. Fortunately, with the excellent and firm but inclusive chairmanship of Ralph Doherty, and the preparedness of the committee's various members to listen to views often vastly different from their own initial opinions or prejudices and to then concede ground where appropriate, the committee functioned extremely well. It helps enormously if members of a committee and its chair can exhibit a sense of humour as well as generosity of spirit, and these features were present in abundance. By coincidence, Bob Smith and Bernie Amos, despite now living far apart, had shared a common experience undertaking national service training decades before and regaled the committee from time to time with their shared experiences.

The process of the inquiry was an exhaustive one, with many submissions received and extensive visits to and consultations with all the existing medical schools. We also visited Darwin and Townsville, which aspired to have medical schools. We learnt a great deal about what was happening in medical education, including recent changes and the frustrations about barriers to change including budget constraints. Attitudes ranged from conservative, with arguments for the preservation of a model of education that its proponents felt had served Australia and the Western world for centuries, to more active, reformist agendas, with problem-based learning or other methodologies espoused.

A particular feature of the inquiry was the holding of 'consumer consultations'. All the relevant consumer organisations in the region were invited to send representatives and the hearings were also more generally open to the public to come and present.

To someone such as me who was committed to a broad and liberal but science-based medical education, these consultations were particularly difficult. The attitude of many of the groups and the people at the meetings was overtly and aggressively hostile to the medical profession and, by extension, to the medical education process which spawned the medical workforce. The pent-up frustration with the system was vented in a manner to which I had not previously been exposed. My initial reaction was defensive and angry when obvious mistruths were expressed and irrational anger was displayed. Clearly, this was an inappropriate reaction, and the greater experience of the chair mostly led to the committee responding to the aggressive assault by patiently listening to the issues raised and responding calmly and unemotionally, thanking the speaker for raising the point.

One notable feature of these consultations was that in very few cases were those who could be reasonably classed as consumers or carers present. Rather than people suffering from chronic disability, epilepsy, diabetes, asthma or whatever, consumer representatives attended and spoke for them, making it harder to accept the exaggerated description of the shortcomings of the profession to which I was so committed.

On one occasion, even the patience of Ralph Doherty, the chair, was stretched beyond breaking point so that his normal patient and bland response was replaced by an ever so slightly adversarial response. On this occasion, the consumer representative had been railing against medical interventions in the birthing process. She made the patently untrue assertion that since doctors had become involved, the rate of maternal and infant death had increased dramatically, quoting an anecdotal source from a small Queensland town. The chair pointed out that the statistics showed exactly the reverse, that is a marked fall in infant and maternal mortality with increased medical involvement in childbirth. This led to the aggressive criticism that we were resorting to the biomedical model relying on statistics and that she rejected that model!

This is an example of a time we felt we were living in parallel universes and that there was no way of reconciling an approach that depended on emotion and anecdote compared with one that depended on what Ralph and I, with our background, would regard as definitive scientific evidence. Our fellow committee members, with their varied backgrounds, were able to calm us down and explain the different perspectives.

We also visited all the medical schools and the universities that aspired to have them and met with many medical craft groups and the Australian Medical Association. One notable surgical specialist group boycotted the process, as there was no representative of their specialty on the committee. We did, however, meet with a senior academic member of that specialty

CHAPTER 11

area. He engaged us in a one-way exposition on how clever his specialty had been in taking his advice on return to this country some decades before. He said that they had 'shut the doors' and that now they were in a position of strength, able, because of their restricted numbers, to dictate employment terms with hospitals and government rebates for services as well as holding a position of great political power and influence. One or two of the more left-wing members of our committee were clearly aghast and this was compounded when he finished his diatribe by saying that 'and there are people on the right wing of our organisation who would say that we did not go far enough'. Given that the medical members of our committee had argued about the altruistic motives of most members of the medical profession and that it was only quality and standards that led to decisions about pass rates and admission of foreign doctors, this was not a particularly helpful, or representative, message.

Overall, the process was a constructive one. From the point of view of medical education, the committee proffered many recommendations arguing for a more student-centred approach to education with active student involvement rather than the traditional didactic approach, more horizontal integration across disciplines and more integration between teaching in the medical sciences and the clinical teaching. It also recommended more attention to population health, preventive approaches to health care and to medicine in rural, remote and Indigenous communities.

Although it was not clear that there was an immediate response to the recommendations concerning medical education, the report served as a blueprint for the guidelines which I later helped to develop as the chair of the accreditation committee of the Australian Medical Council (AMC) about four years later and led to progressive changes to medical education in this country and in view of the extension of the role of the AMC to accrediting medical schools in New Zealand, an influence in that country as well. The medical deans were well aware of the trends in medical education in other countries, but the Doherty Committee Report and the AMC accreditation process helped them to achieve the changes in their faculties that many of the more traditional staff might otherwise have opposed.

The response with respect to the recommendations about the medical workforce was not so immediate. The most important recommendation related to the need to acquire and monitor much better information about the number of doctors practising in Australia and their hours of work. With state-based registration, overlaps between states and difficulty tracking profiles for individual doctors, it was impossible to get accurate data. Moreover, there were disparities between different data sources.

The committee contracted some modelling work based on the projected entry to and exit from the medical workforce. Entry would come from new graduates and migration from overseas, and departures would come from retirement, death or emigration. In contrast to the prevailing opinion at the time, the committee concluded that there would not, at the then current rate of new graduates and migration, be a surfeit of doctors and warned that there could even be a deficit. It did recommend limiting the number of new doctors from overseas to around the current number at the time, which was about 200 per year, although many more came on temporary visas to fill local workforce requirements.

As a result of the recommendation relating to the need for better data, a new committee on which I was asked to sit was established by the commonwealth government with a brief to advise on the acquisition of better workforce data. It was not required to make recommendations on what should be done about the medical workforce one way or the other. This committee, somewhat clumsily named the Medical Workforce Data Review Committee, recommended an annual collection of medical workforce information associated with the state based re-registration process. But given the state control of registration and the fiercely independent nature of some of the medical boards, this was difficult to implement on an Australia-wide basis.

The Medical Workforce Data Review Committee was later replaced by the Australian Medical Workforce Advisory Committee, which reported directly to the Australian Health Ministers Advisory Council, where the chief bureaucrats from the states and commonwealth met together. This was an effective body which made specific recommendations concerning the workforce needs in different medical disciplines. In contrast to the prevailing opinion at the beginning of the 1990s, careful analysis of the data relating to each of the specialties and projections of future demand suggested a need for increased numbers of trainees in virtually all specialties.

Ironically, I was later asked to chair the committee of AMWAC advising on the supply of general practitioners. Using a variety of projections based on trends in working hours and on forecast increased demand associated with ageing of the population, a significant shortfall in the production of general

CHAPTER 11

practitioners was identified. An important consideration was the reduced number of hours that younger doctors were projected to work, partly due to the influence of having a larger percentage of female general practitioners, who on census figures worked on average a third less in their working lives than their male counterparts. Around 700 new general practitioners were being trained each year, whereas the modelling showed a requirement for around 1100 per year to meet demand in ten years.

The medical workforce is always a highly political topic. While the prevailing opinion based on little data in the 1980s was that too many doctors were being produced and that this would lead to excessive costs to Medicare through 'overservicing', this was replaced by data demonstrating a shortfall in the number of doctors in the late 1990s and early in the new century. This has led to an overreaction, with new medical schools and increases in intakes in existing schools causing the number of medical graduates to rise from around 1400 in the mid 1990s to about 3000 by 2012. Once steady-state is established, there will be an oversupply of doctors as assessed by conventional measures of need, and the cycle may well be repeated.

A particularly sensitive area for governments is the supply of doctors to rural areas. In Australia, as in other countries with relatively vast and underpopulated areas away from capital cities, it is difficult to attract sufficient doctors to rural areas. This has been the subject of numerous enquiries and policies attempting to redress the problem.

The simplest is to graduate more doctors, hoping for a 'trickle down' effect.

Although this may occur to some extent, our fee-for-service, publicly funded private system, combined with the ability of both doctors and patients to rationalise increased services in already well-served metropolitan regions, means that relying on this mechanism is slow and inefficient.

A variety of carrots relating to employment conditions have been and continue to be used with some effect. Threats to restrict the supply of 'provider numbers', which are necessary for doctors to access Medicare, have not been followed through for Australian graduates, but such restrictions have been applied to for doctors from overseas.

A very positive initiative of Michael Wooldridge when he was minister for health in the Howard government was to establish departments of rural health and rural clinical schools with new funding and a requirement for a large proportion of medical students to have a significant period of their clinical training in rural locations. These have proved very successful, with students becoming very enthusiastic about their rural experience and a number of charismatic teachers inspiring many students to return to rural practice, at least for a period of their careers. The students found that the range of clinical conditions they saw and the enthusiasm for patients to engage with students were greater than in the large teaching hospitals in the cities. In the city hospitals, pressure on hospital beds and the highly specialised nature of many of the units made it difficult for students to spend time with patients with common conditions that they needed to learn about.

Another positive initiative was the introduction of rural scholarships. Students could opt for scholarships which provided living allowances and exemption from fees in exchange for a commitment to spend six years in rural areas or other areas of need during or immediately after their hospital training period. This voluntary system was well received.

In contrast, a later scheme to add extra medical school places provided that the recipients were prepared to commit to a similar period in rural areas or other defined areas of workforce need was ill conceived and caused great resentment amongst the medical student community. The inference to be drawn from this program was clear. Rural practice was only for those forced to do it because they could not gain entry to an unencumbered medical school place. This was exactly the reverse of the very positive message given from the wonderful experiences that most students experienced in their rural clinical schools. Two steps forward and one step backwards!

The medical workforce will always remain a difficult issue. Within our Medicare system, we cannot rely on market forces to lead to students responding to supply and demand to regulate intake. Unfortunately, political pressures often lead to decisions designed to satisfy a short-term problem without taking account of long-term consequences.

Chapter 12

THE MEDICAL SCHOOL ACCREDITATION COMMITTEE OF THE AUSTRALIAN MEDICAL COUNCIL

After a lot of discussion about the need for an independent national standards body for medical education and training, the AMC was finally established by the commonwealth government in 1984. Initially, it was assigned three functions.

The first was to accredit medical schools in Australia and later in New Zealand. The second was the assessment of overseas trained medical practitioners to determine their suitability and eligibility for practice in Australia. The third was to progress towards uniform standards and practices for medical registration and disciplinary procedures between the states. In 2000, additional functions, the accreditation of the training and assessment processes of the medical specialties and the provision of advice to the federal government on the registration of new specialties, were added to the roles of the AMC.

The AMC was comprised of presidents of state and territory medical boards, the chairs of the medical schools accreditation committee and the examinations committee for foreign medical graduates, and nominees from the state and commonwealth departments of health via the Australian Health Ministers Advisory Council, universities and postgraduate education committees. There have been modifications to its structure and function over time, and the establishment by the commonwealth of the National Registration and Accreditation Scheme will significantly reduce the role of the AMC with respect to its function as an umbrella organisation for the regulatory boards in the states and territories. Its key roles in accreditation of medical schools, medical specialist assessment and training and advising on new medical specialties will remain and, it is to be hoped, will serve as a model for regulatory structures for the other health professions. In 2008, for the first time, the president was not one of the presidents of a medical board from one of the states or territories but the chair of the Specialist Education Accreditation Committee, Professor Dick Smallwood.

I was asked to join the Medical School Accreditation Committee of the AMC in 1990 and held the position of chair of this committee from 1991 to 1995. The initial chair had been Professor John Hamilton, the dean of the Faculty of Health Sciences at the University of Newcastle in New South Wales.

Both the need for the committee and the nature of the process were highly controversial at the time of their establishment. It was also questioned whether the process would have any teeth. The first medical school to be assessed was the University of Queensland. A number of problems were identified which had to be addressed before full accreditation was granted some time later. This at least showed that the process would not automatically grant unconditional accreditation to medical schools, even if they were long established and with a high reputation.

An apocryphal tale (not necessarily untrue) quoted the University of Melbourne's vice-chancellor David Penington as saying at his opening and supposedly welcoming meeting with the assessment team from the AMC shortly after the Queensland assessment that he would like the team to realise that it was the AMC, not the University of Melbourne's medical school, that was on trial!

When I commenced as chair, a major task was to produce local guidelines for use by the Accreditation Committee and by universities and medical schools to guide them towards what was expected of the schools. Up until then, the guidelines developed by the General Medical Council of the UK had been used.

The task in preparing new guidelines was to ensure a balance between two potentially conflicting requirements. The first was to ensure that they were sufficiently detailed and specific to reassure the medical boards of the various states and territories which used accreditation by the AMC as the basis for determining whether the graduates were registrable as doctors. The second was to allow enough leeway to encourage innovation in medical education. The approach was to emphasise graduate attributes containing

CHAPTER 12

some key components of knowledge, skills and attitudes, rather than prescribing curricula or teaching methods. Medical schools were required to indicate how they ensured, through their curriculum, teaching methods and assessments, that their graduates had attained the required attributes.

The guidelines emphasised a number of topic areas which had been identified by the Doherty Committee as having not received sufficient attention in medical schools. These included rural medicine, preventive medicine, Indigenous health, cross-cultural competence and communication techniques. Emphasis was also placed on involving students more actively as active learners, rather than as rote learners, and in discovering information themselves.

After a period of discussion and modification, the guidelines were introduced and served as the basis for the accreditation process. They have undergone modifications but still serve to guide the development of new medical schools, major modifications of existing schools and reaccreditation of established schools.

Given the sensitivity of the assessment process for overseas trained medical practitioners, there has been pressure from time to time to replace the accreditation process with a single national qualifying examination applying to both local graduates and to overseas-trained graduates as a requirement for registration for practice in Australia. Although this has the advantage of a common requirement for Australian and foreign graduates and therefore removes any perception of prejudice against foreign graduates, I was and remain opposed to the concept.

The assessment process drives the learning techniques and methods of students. Medical schools in Australia have evolved complex longitudinal methods of assessment which are aligned with the objectives of the educational process. Continuing assessment in the wards and on placements are important parts of this assessment, so the students assign these tasks the importance they deserve. Detailed evaluation of clinical competence using a variety of assessment methods is applied. Hurdles are set along the way to assure the medical school, the registration boards and the public of the competence of the graduates. These assessments could not be performed in a similar way at a single point in time on a national basis.

Our medical schools have been innovative and creative in developing individual curricula and pedagogical approaches which have satisfied the accreditation guidelines and also demonstrated diversity. A single national qualifying examination would undoubtedly lessen the diversity, as students would expect their educational experience to be directed towards acquiring the knowledge to satisfy the examination. Practical considerations would make it difficult to assess fairly and adequately skills and attitudes on a national basis.

Ideally, foreign graduates would undergo longitudinal assessment of knowledge, skills and attitudes in a manner similar to local graduates, and the introduction of more diverse methods of assessment through specialist colleges has moved the assessment of a significant proportion of foreign graduates in this direction.

Although the absence of a national qualifying examination exposes the AMC and the medical boards to accusations of bias against foreign graduates on the one hand or laxity in accepting the qualifications of incompetent doctors on the other hand, the adverse effects of introducing a common system for local and foreign graduates would outweigh the benefits.

After the initial suspicion, the accreditation process has become accepted and respected. Medical deans recognise that it gives them a powerful tool to modernise curricula, to improve quality of education and to gain greater cooperation from state governments, hospitals and divisions of general practice in supporting medical education. On a number of occasions, accreditation was granted only for a limited period with a requirement to address major problems that had been identified. By and large, medical schools were able to address the problems identified, often achieving greater support from their universities or hospitals and on review they could usually achieve full accreditation.

The New Zealand Medical Council had no process for accrediting its medical schools and asked whether it could join the AMC process. This was agreed. I led the assessment team to the University of Otago. The team was largely made up of members with diverse backgrounds in medical education from Australia, but it also included the dean of the Faculty of Medical and Health Sciences from the University of Auckland, Peter Gluckman. We felt there might be some sensitivity about the process. After all, depending on 'big brother' from Australia to say whether medical education at the old and much revered University of Otago was up to scratch could well be resented.

In the event, the process was quite tense. But the real sensitivity was not directed to the Australian members of the team, but instead to the 'dean

CHAPTER 12

from the north', who was viewed, at least by some, with suspicion bordering on paranoia.

The process at that time included a final verbal report to the school giving an indication of the findings of the team, although not actually announcing the decision about accreditation. The responsibility for the final decision lay with the full council of the AMC, which made its recommendation to the New Zealand Medical Council.

The delivery of the report was a highly charged affair. Not only was the lecture theatre at the headquarters of the medical school in Dunedin full, but the delivery was video-cast to equally full lecture theatres at the two additional clinical schools of the University of Otago medical school in Wellington and Christchurch. There were a number of issues that the team was concerned about, including the organisational structure of the faculty, which was cumbersome, the funding available to the school from the university and the government and recent decisions about support (or lack of it) for medical research by the Health Research Council and government.

The executive dean, who had been directly involved in all these aspects, was the endocrinologist David Stewart. He and his wife, Doff, had been charming hosts and entertained our whole family at his summer house when he invited me as the guest lecturer to the Endocrine Society of New Zealand ten years before. The criticisms that I conveyed on behalf of my team all seemed to be directed towards him and his several roles in government and on the Health Research Council as well as in the university. He must have felt it was a poor way to repay the previous hospitality. As always, he was a total gentleman, accepting the criticisms constructively, and the University of Otago responded positively to the recommendations.

My role as the chair of the Accreditation Committee led to my serving on the executive of the AMC. At that time, it was heavily embroiled in legal challenges from disaffected foreign medical graduates challenging the imposition of a quota and its examination procedures and alleging bias. It was a difficult time for the AMC, but it led to a careful review of its processes and it emerged stronger.

After completing four years as chair of the Medical School Accreditation Committee, I left the AMC convinced that it was performing a valuable role. I returned briefly some years later as the chair of the Specialist Education Accreditation Committee, which was charged with the new function of accrediting the training and examination methods of the specialist colleges but resigned when I took up the vice-chancellorship of Monash University in 2003.

Although these processes often cause resentment as a bureaucratic intrusion into the autonomy and independence of medical schools and colleges, I believe that they are necessary processes to reassure the public and the medical boards about the quality of the medical practitioners and specialists being produced. As they depend on a peer review process and are conducted in a collegial way, they are as 'light touch' as they could be while performing their function of assuring quality. They are now well accepted, and as the commonwealth government moves towards a national system of accreditation and registration of health professions, the AMC process is being held up as a model for other health professions.

Chapter 13

DEPUTY DEAN OF THE FACULTY OF MEDICINE, DENTISTRY AND HEALTH SCIENCES AT THE UNIVERSITY OF MELBOURNE, AND REFORM OF THE MEDICAL CURRICULUM

In 1995, shortly after Alan Gilbert had been announced as the successor to David Penington as vice-chancellor of the University of Melbourne, the dean of the Faculty of Medicine, Dentistry and Health Sciences, Graeme Ryan, announced that he was resigning to take up the position of CEO of St Vincent's Hospital. I was approached by a number of members of the faculty to sound out my interest in becoming dean. I was not ready to do so at that stage. I had just had surgery for carcinoma of the bladder, and in addition, Caroline and I had planned to take long-service leave combined with the Sir Arthur Simms Commonwealth Travelling Professorship, which had been awarded to me by the Royal College of Surgeons and the Royal College of Physicians of London. This would entail three months travelling through Canada, the UK, Sri Lanka and Malaysia delivering lectures and making visits related to my diabetes research and also learning of advances in medical education. I did not feel I could assume the deanship and shortly after take-off for three months. I therefore indicated that I would not be available at that time, although should the position come up at some time in the future, I may well be.

My colleague Gordon Clunie was duly appointed. Gordon was the James Stewart Professor of Surgery at the Royal Melbourne Hospital, and we had been close colleagues in advancing the cause of the university within the hospital. As Gordon was approaching retirement, some felt that he might occupy something of a caretaker role rather than being actively reformist.

In fact, he was very active in the two years in which he occupied the position. He, like me, recognised the need to undertake a major revision of the medical education program of the university. There had been some change during the deanship of David Penington over a decade before, with more teaching of family medicine and population health, more integration of preclinical and clinical sciences, but essentially, the pedagogical approaches and much of the content of the educational process were unchanged from the time I had been a student.

The attitude was that the course was producing excellent graduates, and the medical school was recognised around the world as being of high quality. Many of the academic staff had international reputations in research and did not have the appetite for or see the need for a major change in the curriculum or approach to teaching and learning. Moreover, Graeme Ryan had been fully engaged with and very effective at enlarging the faculty by bringing in the dental school, a step resented by much of the dental profession but very necessary for the viability of the school and commencing a school of physiotherapy. A school of postgraduate nursing had also been established and was about to commence teaching.

The AMC had accredited the school with comments along the lines that it was a traditional medical school which was carrying out this traditional approach well. Although there was no immediate threat from the AMC, both Gordon and I felt that with the changes being undertaken in medical education throughout the Western world, the university could not rely on its reputation in the next round of the accreditation process. It really had to undertake the hard task of major reform of the medical curriculum and mode of teaching. Gordon appointed me as deputy dean and the planning dean, with a major responsibility for planning a new curriculum. These were part-time appointments while I continued as professor of medicine and head of a general medical unit at the Royal Melbourne Hospital. I had handed over the directorship of the department of diabetes and endocrinology, which I had taken up on Skip Martin's retirement, to Peter Colman, but I continued to have clinical responsibilities in that discipline as well as in general medicine and my half day a week of private practice. It was a busy time and as happens in those situations, it was research time that was most squeezed. I was fortunate

CHAPTER 13

in having Marjorie Dunlop performing an outstanding role in the laboratory, along with a number of postdoctoral colleagues and research students.

During my tenure of the Simms Travelling Professorship, I visited a number of medical schools which had undertaken radical reform of their curricula. I spent particular time with the University of British Columbia in Vancouver, Calgary University, the University of Toronto, McMaster University, Ottawa University and McGill University. McMaster had been the pioneer in problem-based learning (PBL), with the University of Newcastle in Australia being an early adopter. The Canadian universities I visited had all embraced this to varying extents, with Calgary being the most extreme.

The theory of PBL is that students should be actively engaged in the education process. Information sought out by students to solve the problem that they are confronting will be better remembered. Moreover, as the information has been learnt in the context of a clinical problem, the students can more readily apply this to the clinical situations they confront. This method of learning is also more engaging for students compared with passive involvement in listening to lectures.

There are now many variants of PBL, but in essence the students are assigned to groups of ten or so, and there is progressive unfolding of a (usually) clinical scenario. At stages along the evolution of the scenario, the students analyse the questions that are raised by it. For example, if the initial problem relates to a patient passing blood in their urine and this is at a very early stage in their course, they might start by asking about the possible sources of the blood, which would lead to one of the group being assigned the task of going through the anatomy of the urinary tract and kidneys. Then, it is necessary to understand how urine is formed, so someone else might be asked to study this question. Then the question of potential pathological or disease processes that could lead to blood in the urine would be examined. The students meet as a group two or three times on a single problem, usually over a period of a week. Of course, expectations of students at the start of their medical course and of those approaching the end of their course would be quite different.

Tutors are trained to help the students determine the boundaries of their enquiries and not to provide the factual content, which the students must learn for themselves. In addition to encouraging the students in research and discovery, the approach also helps the students to work in teams and to communicate – vital skills in all professions and certainly in medicine.

There are unquestionable advantages to this form of pedagogy. But there are also some weaknesses. Although it does provide integration of the basic medical sciences with clinical medicine, it cuts across the integration of the specific disciplines. There is a logic and coherence about the biochemical systems operating in different body systems, the anatomical structures throughout the body and the physiological processes determining their function. It is hard for the students to get a comprehensive view of these systems. They are not confined to a specific part of the body involved in an individual disease, and it is therefore difficult to get a concept of the overall system from the study of a particular problem.

It is also difficult for students to gain a concept of what they do not know – in the words immortalised by Donald Rumsfeld, the 'unknown unknowns'. This gives some students a sense of insecurity. This insecurity is greatest early in the course, where so many new concepts are broached that the students cannot follow up each of them adequately. It is the tutors' task to reassure the students that there will be many opportunities later in the course to return to some of these concepts, but it is still difficult to circumscribe the knowledge and understanding expected at each stage.

With time, these issues have been addressed to a considerable extent. For example, the design of a new curriculum requires a map to be established indicating the knowledge, skills and attitudes required at the completion of the course and where in the course these particular attributes will be acquired.

Some medical schools have attempted to adhere to the PBL approach as the exclusive or almost-exclusive method of education. In 1996, when I did my tour, the medical school at the University of Calgary was following this approach most completely. Their medical course offered only to graduates was only three years in length, but the years were long and intensive, so that the number of teaching (learning) weeks was about the same as the four-year graduate courses.

Most of the medical schools I visited had attempted to provide a more definite structure to the program by combining PBL with lectures of one type or another (however styled) and practical sessions. The lectures are designed to provide the students with help in gaining understanding of some difficult concepts and ideally do not cover the same topics as those

CHAPTER 13

addressed by the problems. Even the pioneers of PBL, such as McMaster University in Canada, Maastricht University in Holland and the University of Newcastle in Australia, have moved away from a purist PBL-based program to a more hybrid curriculum. This addresses some of the difficulties in a PBL-alone program, including the different learning styles and preferences of individual students, and makes the overall program more varied and interesting.

In addition to changes in the methods of teaching, there was also an urgent need to address the content of the program. Over the years, there had been a vast increase in knowledge, most notably derived from understanding the genetic code and the huge power of molecular biology. This led to the need for students to understand the principles of genomics and the new investigative techniques which were being applied increasingly in clinical medicine. More and more information was being added to the curriculum and nothing was being dropped off.

Moreover, although there had been attempts to alter this, there was too much time spent on uncommon diseases in metropolitan teaching hospitals and too little time spent on population health, preventive medicine, general practice, international health, legal aspects of medicine and medical ethics, to name a few disciplines. This would require a major reorganisation of curriculum content, with a significant reduction in content of some of the traditional components to make way for the new. For example, it is hard to justify 260 hours of dissection of cadavers. Many medical schools have totally done away with student dissection and instead have the students study plastinated specimens already dissected or layered 3D computer images. The content of traditional biochemistry must also be reduced.

It is not difficult to understand that academics who are experts in these fields, and have dedicated their lives to their study and to transmitting their knowledge to successive generations of students, regret and in some cases vigorously contest the reduction in content of their discipline and its disintegration through an approach that is based on integrating all disciplines around individual body systems, such the cardiovascular system or the gastrointestinal system.

By the mid-1990s, technology was starting to have a big impact on all forms of education, and medical schools were taking a lead role. The PBL program lent itself well to presentation in a computer format with progressive unfolding of information during the course of the week in which the problem was being studied. But in addition, carefully designed programs could be constructed and delivered either online or via CDs to address difficult areas of the curriculum. It is important that these programs actively involve the students and are not merely electronic textbooks. This requires creativity so that the program is truly interactive, with the students needing to discover and apply knowledge. By interspersing evaluation of the students' knowledge and comparing this to the class mean, a valuable form of feedback to the student can be provided. Feedback is an area which the students frequently identify as the weakest area when evaluation of their satisfaction with a particular subject is undertaken.

It was clear to me on my visits to medical schools around the world that there was much that we needed to do in Melbourne. Gordon Clunie was of the same mind, but the medical school faculty were far from convinced at that stage that anything apart from some fine-tuning was required. Moreover, for the valid reasons stated above, some were strongly opposed. As with all medical schools contemplating radical change, it was necessary to convince the faculty that this was not only desirable, but necessary.

An off-site retreat was convened by Gordon Clunie and a heated but constructive debate on the pros and cons of a move towards an integrated course with PBL featuring prominently, although not as the sole method of pedagogy.

It was also necessary to resolve whether to move to a graduate-entry program, which was the norm in North America and had been adopted at Flinders University, the University of Queensland and University of Sydney. Arguments for this model included the greater maturity of graduates compared with school leavers, which would allow a more mature selection of career and a more focused approach to their education. The undergraduate course, if it was not focused on life sciences, would provide students with a broader education than one focused only on medicine. It was also argued that there was a better basis for selection at the graduate level, including students' undergraduate performance, an interview and a specifically designed graduate medical school admissions assessment already tested and apparently performing well. Graduate level selection could also compensate in part for the difficulty for students in rural areas and underperforming secondary schools to achieve the required high school certificate level for undergraduate entry, making selection more equitable.

CHAPTER 13

Against this, there are also arguments in favour of direct entry to medical school from secondary school. For example, for those students who are convinced they wish to study medicine and who have demonstrated by their high school results that they are capable of completing the course satisfactorily, it is frustrating to have to undertake another course that may not interest them and then to compete for entry once more. The idea that the undergraduate course provides breadth is contradicted by the high proportion of students undertaking courses in biological sciences as a prelude to applying for graduate medical school (most such schools would have well over 80 per cent of students with a biological or health science background). The total duration of university study is prolonged from five or six years to seven years, with associated extra expense for the student and for the government. And the medical course itself is shortened from six to four years, with less opportunity to undertake research, additional diplomas (for example, music or a foreign language) or to take a gap year before or during the course.

There is also a more pragmatic reason for selecting at least some of the students directly from secondary school. Each medical school likes to get its share (or more) of the brightest students. Although high school examination results might be only one measure of the likelihood of a student performing well at university and even less a predictor of a successful research career, it does seem courageous for a medical school to design an entry process which might encourage the best performing high school students to choose another university offering direct entry. The University of Melbourne's medical school had already benefitted from this, with quite a large number of the best-performing school leavers in Queensland choosing to come to the medical school at the University of Melbourne, which offered them a definite place and allowed them to commence medical studies at once. The other medical school in Melbourne at that time, Monash University, showed no intention of moving to graduate entry, and we had no wish to see Monash become the preferred destination for the best-performing would-be medical students.

After much debate on the pros and cons of graduate entry, the faculty decided on a novel composite model. Two-thirds of the students would enter directly from school and undertake a five-year medical course but would also be required to choose from a variety of options for an additional intercalated year after two and a half years of their medical course. Most students would do a year of research. The fields for this research could vary from laboratory science related to medicine or the preclinical disciplines through to population health, humanities or social sciences related to medicine, including the history of medicine, medicine and law, ethics and so on. Satisfactory completion of this year would lead to a second degree, a Bachelor of Medical Science. Some students who had chosen to do a combined degree with arts would be able to do a concentrated year of arts, allowing them to complete combined MBBS and BA degrees in seven years, which was possible only with significant overloading of the students' teaching commitments with the existing six-year medical course.

It was agreed, reluctantly by some, to adopt a change in pedagogy to a largely PBL-based format with a limited number of lectures and a totally revised program of practical classes which would emphasise clinically relevant aspects of physiology and in some cases biochemistry, pharmacology and anatomy. Clinical medicine and some contact with patients would be introduced from the beginning of the course (vertical integration), and there would be integration of the preclinical sciences around body systems and clinical problems (horizontal integration). Contact hours would be markedly reduced from about thirty hours per week to around eighteen or twenty to allow more time for self-directed learning, including computer-based learning from the internet and CDs. Teaching in the hospitals and general practice would also change to become more integrated around body systems rather than the haphazard approach used up to that time, where it was hoped that the major systems were covered and gaps might be filled by a lecture series.

One third of the students would be graduates from other courses. Students with a biomedical science background would be exempted from the first semester and instead given a bridging program immediately before commencing second semester. Students without a biomedical science background would start at the commencement of the first semester with the undergraduate-entry students. The graduate-entry cohort would then study with the undergraduates until the completion of semester five, when they would not be required to undertake the research (Bachelor of Medical Science) year and would then join the cohort of undergraduate students from the previous year's intake, who would be returning from their Bachelor of Medical Science year and starting the phase of the course based largely in hospitals and general practice. The graduates would

CHAPTER 13

therefore complete their course in four and a half years for those with a biomedical background or five years for those without.

It should be noted that clinical teaching at its best was already problem-based. The patient presents with a problem, and the history and examination of the patient is designed to sort that out. A good tutor would take the students through the steps in clinical problem-solving and it was hoped that the background of the students in PBL in the earlier phases of the course would better prepare the students for their clinical experience. It is recognised that while it is easy to bring clinical facets of a problem into the early parts of a medical course, it is much harder to keep the basic medical science aspects prominent in the later parts of the course, where most students are seduced by the clinical features without reprising the basic aspects. Introducing structured problems into this part of the course was designed to achieve this, although it is difficult to sustain the students' interest in these exercises in the frenetic atmosphere of a teaching hospital or general practice.

Most traditional medical textbooks at the time were organised around diseases, but most patients present complaining of problems such as shortness of breath, pain in various sites, nausea and vomiting, tiredness, dizziness or a variety of other symptoms. Recognising this, Professor Priscilla Kincaid-Smith, head of nephrology and a valued senior colleague in the department of medicine at the Royal Melbourne Hospital, asked me and Professor Greg Whelan, a gastroenterologist based at St Vincent's Hospital who had a particular interest and background in medical education, to join her in editing and contributing to a textbook based around the approach to patients' presenting problems. Shortly after this, Professor Richard Smallwood from the Austin Hospital and I also wrote a book on clinical history and examination as a successor to Lovell and Doyle's clinical guide that we had used as students. It had stood us in good stead but was now a little outmoded in style.

Our book on clinical history and examination was based on the more recent approach of basing the clinical history and examination on identifying and solving the patient's problems rather than a systematic scan of each system. Systematic questioning and other aspects of family history or past history were used as safety nets to pick up unsuspected aspects which may not have been revealed by following up the patient's presenting and additional self-identified problems. These two books were well suited to the new curriculum, and their preparation also helped to clarify my own approach to medical education.

Next, the issue of selection had to be addressed. We decided that for the one third of students coming in as graduates, the method used by the other graduate-entry schools would be followed. A combination of the grade point average (GPA) in the undergraduate course, performance in the Graduate Australian Medical School Admissions Test (GAMSAT), which had been developed in combination with the Australian Council for Educational Research (ACER), and a structured interview for candidates performing well on GPA and GAMSAT was settled on.

For undergraduates, it was more difficult. It could be argued that the performance in the final secondary school examinations, in Victoria the Victorian Certificate of Education, would serve as a good index of the combination of commitment and intelligence. However, if this alone were to be used, almost all the students would come from elite independent schools and selective entry government high schools. On the basis of the Equivalent National Tertiary Education Rank (ENTER), only very occasional students from rural and suburban high schools record a rank above the ninety-ninth percentile, which is required if this is the only criterion on which entry to medicine is decided. Already, the commonwealth government had placed a benchmark that 25 per cent of entrants to medical school should have a rural background, justifying a separate selection pool for these students. But we did not feel that this sufficiently addressed the necessity of admitting students with a variety of backgrounds and providing students from a less-advantaged socio-economic background with a reasonable opportunity of studying medicine as undergraduates.

Several medical schools use structured interview as one of the criteria for assessing entrance to medical schools. Indeed, we had decided we would do this for the graduate-entry stream. However, we felt that using an interview at school-leaver level would do little to address the disadvantage that students from less privileged educational backgrounds face. Students from independent schools with parents in the professions are more likely to be articulate and to be able to verbalise why they wish to study medicine than students who are the first generation in their families to go to university, who are educated in the tough environment of high schools in low socio-economic areas and often have a non-English speaking background. Moreover, it is difficult to use interview to assess suitability for the wide variety of careers

CHAPTER 13

that medical graduates follow. I often used as examples of the frailty of the interview process two individuals. One was Sir Frank Macfarlane Burnet, who was awarded the Nobel Prize in Physiology or Medicine. He was a shy man who found it difficult to look people in the eye while speaking to them and who I am sure would not have performed well in a structured interview over thirty minutes. The second was a medical school contemporary of mine who was extremely engaging, intelligent and articulate and who would have scored very highly in any interview. He spent his career engaging in any entrepreneurial activity likely to earn a lot of money and was ultimately debarred from medical practice by the medical boards of New South Wales and Victoria. Anecdotes do not make an argument and I apologise for resorting to them.

The Undergraduate Medical and Health Professions Admission Test (UMAT) had been devised by the Australian Council for Educational Research to address this issue. It consisted of three parts. The first was a test of logic and problem-solving. The second was designed to test empathy, communication and ethical decision-making. The third was designed to test non-verbal intelligence. Theoretically at least, the test was not dependent on practice or preparation for the test.

Initially, we proposed that a composite of the ENTER ranking and the UMAT ranking would be used. After the first year, we had complaints from students and their teachers which were compelling. Students who received the very top percentile ranking (99.95) had been rejected on the basis of their UMAT scores. Fine, this is what a composite score was meant to achieve – a blending of academic achievement and other attributes not measured in the final secondary school examinations. But school principals then indicated that some of the students excluded on the basis of the UMAT score, despite the highest possible ENTER, were clearly outstanding individuals in every respect – sometimes school captains, members of school debating teams, performing many voluntary and worthy activities and voted by their classmates as the most popular students in the school.

After this, we modified the selection criteria for undergraduate students, so that 25 per cent of students were selected on the basis of their ENTER rank, provided their UMAT was above the twentieth percentile, 25 per cent were selected on the basis of their UMAT score, provided that their ENTER was above the ninety-sixth percentile (lower for rural students and students from socio-economically disadvantaged backgrounds), and 50 per cent were selected from a composite of the ENTER and the UMAT. This recognised that students obtaining very high ENTERs had some special attributes as did students with the very highest UMAT rankings. Given that 33 per cent of students were selected as graduates on different criteria, and special processes or dispensations were used for rural and Indigenous students, we felt that we had arrived at as fair a process as is possible in the highly fraught situation where many more able and committed students wish to study medicine than there are available places.

I believed that the composite model of undergraduate and graduate entry served the University of Melbourne well for the thirteen years it was operating. Many students who would otherwise not have had any contact with research became genuinely enthused by it, and the university departments and medical research institutes receiving such students appreciated the opportunity of engaging with such intelligent students at a formative stage of their medical education. With the move of the University of Melbourne entirely to graduate entry for medicine and other professional degrees in 2012, the blended model has been superseded. Given that biomedical science is to be a prerequisite, it does seem to be a reversion to separate preclinical and clinical education in a total period of seven years in a less integrated fashion than had been achieved, although I know there will be many innovations and improvements in the graduate-entry course.

Chapter 14

DEAN OF THE FACULTY OF MEDICINE, DENTISTRY AND HEALTH SCIENCES AT THE UNIVERSITY OF MELBOURNE

At the end of 1997, Gordon Clunie retired as the dean of the Faculty of Medicine, Dentistry and Health Sciences (MDHS) at the University of Melbourne. He had done an outstanding job in the two years he was dean following the resignation of Graeme Ryan. As described in chapter 13, he had initiated the most extensive reform of medical education ever seen at the University of Melbourne and navigated some treacherous waters at meetings of the faculty board.

This board was large, with extensive representation from the professions outside the university. To demonstrate the difficulties Gordon encountered, he proposed that the name of the medical degree be changed from its traditional Bachelor of Medicine and Bachelor of Surgery (MBBS) to the more generic MB (Bachelor of Medicine). Although 'medicine' was being used to describe the discipline at large, and reflected the fact that just as the specialty areas of internal medicine and surgery might have some claim to appear in the name of the degree, so too might obstetrics and gynaecology, paediatrics, general practice, pathology and public health – clearly a nonsense. Moreover, designating the new course with a new title would signal its radical (for the University of Melbourne) nature.

The objective of changing its name was seen as a conspiracy and boisterously opposed by two sections of the faculty board. One vocal member, a general practitioner, argued that it was a deliberate attempt by surgeons such as the dean to prevent general practitioners from undertaking any form of surgery. Some surgeons on the board on the other hand saw it as an attempt to marginalise the discipline of surgery in the educational program and to make it subservient to medicine!

In the event, Gordon and I decided not to push the point and prejudice the acceptance of the new course by controversies surrounding its name. It was a big enough task to encourage the preclinical disciplines to give up some of their teaching time and a considerable degree of the control of their discipline's curriculum and to support the new integrated curriculum without getting sidetracked by something so trivial as the name of the degree.

The detailed design of the new course occurred in 1998, with the objective of introducing it in 1999. It was a frenetic period, overseen by the new Faculty Education Unit, led by an admirable young gastroenterologist, Susan Elliott. The tens of working parties and the hundreds of members of these working parties did an outstanding job in the detailed design of the new curriculum, ensuring that they were able to map the identified topics that needed to be covered in themes of the curriculum. Some topics would be addressed in the problems which were to form the nucleus of the learning modalities, others in the reduced number of lectures, practical classes and interactive multimedia resources. Although many learning tools were becoming available on the net and in commercially available CDs, their quality and relevance were not thought sufficient for our purposes. Moreover, participation in the design and preparation of new resources 'homemade' by the faculty would give a degree of ownership and pride that would lead to more people being infected with the passion for medical education in general and for the new curriculum in particular. This was overseen by the medical multimedia unit outstandingly led by a physiologist, Peter Harris, who had a particular passion for the area.

A new requirement was for problem-based learning (PBL) tutors. As described in chapter 13, responsibility for providing these was allocated to academic departments determined by the difference in the funding they received for education and their contribution to the 'set pieces' in the new compared with the old curriculum. These tutors required a specific training program. Many experienced teachers found the need to let the students explore possibilities with minimal intervention from the tutors very frustrating, and some could not achieve the conversion from the role of active teacher to the much more passive role of PBL 'facilitator'. Some of the new PBL tutors were PhD students. Their scholarships allowed them some time for outside work, and the teaching experience was valuable for them in

CHAPTER 14

relation to their later career choices. Of course, they, like all the other tutors, had to undertake the PBL training program.

A novel feature of the course was the compulsory 'Advanced Medical Sciences' or AMS year that all the undergraduate students, with the exception of those doing a combined medicine and arts degree, were required to take. The combined course students could do a year of their arts program instead. A variety of research options were approved for this year, ranging from basic laboratory-based biomedical science in one of the university's departments or in an affiliated research institute to humanities- or social science-based research and scholarship relevant to medicine such as medical ethics, history of medicine and legal aspects of medicine. Provided that the proposed program fulfilled the defined requirements of the year, it could also be taken overseas.

Initially, many students chose an option in anatomy, which provided an opportunity to do more dissection. Although there were worthwhile research objectives, many students chose this option because they were concerned that their exposure to anatomy may have been reduced too dramatically and that unless they did more anatomy, they might not be able to become surgeons. Gradually, this anxiety dissipated and students chose electives according to their interests, word of mouth from the experience of previous students and the enthusiasm of the host department or institute in promoting their option.

By and large, this year was a great success. Many students did very worthwhile research, with publications and presentations resulting. The students mostly enjoyed the year very much and appreciated the insights into research and scholarship. I do not know how many chose an academic or research career as a result of this experience, but it certainly raised this possibility in the minds of many who would not otherwise have contemplated such a career. The departments and institutes which hosted such students found it a very positive experience, as the students were generally highly intelligent, motivated and productive.

An area where the faculty was strong but in which it had a limited profile outside the university was in public health and epidemiology. There were many strong individual researchers and groups in the different departments and schools of the faculty. I thought that the only way to increase the effectiveness of this area of health education and research was to bring all the researchers together in a geographic or virtual sense. After many meetings, the School of Population Health was formed to sit alongside the School of Medicine, School of Dental Science and School of Physiotherapy and Nursing. Under the leadership of Terry Nolan, it became a very strong and visible centre for public health and epidemiology research and education.

The faculty had indeed become complex. In terms of staff numbers, budgets and research output, the School of Medicine was by far the largest school in the faculty. My role combined the roles of dean of the Faculty of Medicine, Dentistry and Health Sciences with that of head of the School of Medicine. This had the disadvantage that the other schools could feel that my role as both dean and head of one of the schools was conflicted. It also meant that it was a very big job. On the other hand, in those universities where the role of dean has been separated from that of head of the School of Medicine, both the dean's role and the head of the medical school's roles are difficult. The dean is not in direct control of the dominant school, the budget and research productivity of which determines, to a significant extent, the success of the faculty and indeed the whole university. On the other hand, the head of the School of Medicine often does not have control of his or her budget and, given the importance of the school to the faculty, often has to put up with significant interference or at least ambiguity of responsibilities with the dean. I think the model we had while I was dean worked for me and the faculty. But to make it work, we had to be more than fair to the smaller schools – this had little impact on the School of Medicine but made a large difference to the smaller schools.

Another initiative funded by the federal government, under the leadership of the minister for health Michael Wooldridge, was the establishment initially of departments of rural health and later rural clinical schools. Ours was based in Shepparton. After a chequered start, where it was difficult to attract medical students and some problems with the initial staffing of the school, it has become extremely popular with the students under the leadership of Dawn DeWitt, whom I recruited from the United States. Dawn was a charismatic individual, who quickly inspired the students to come and discover the pleasure of studying and later working in a rural environment.

An earlier head of the school, David Simmons, had established a relationship with the Indigenous community in Shepparton and, in partnership with local Indigenous leader Paul Briggs and the Rumbalara Football and Netball Club, had started an Academy of Sport Health and Education

CHAPTER 14

(ASHE). The idea was that by engaging Indigenous secondary school students through their passionate interest in sport, that entry point could be used to strengthen their sense of cultural pride and progressively to deliver health messages, educational support and vocational training programs. This initiative has been transferred to the Faculty of Education and has been successful.

Vice-Chancellor Alan Gilbert attended the launch of the Rural Clinical School by Prime Minister John Howard. In the euphoria of the moment, Alan promised that Shepparton would become a university town of the University of Melbourne and offered AUS$5 million to help this happen. The Rural Clinical School remains the only substantial evidence of this initiative, but indeed this has been a most successful development.

The dental school was the site of significant unrest at that time. There was a major rift between the school's head and a recently arrived professor, and it was dividing the school. Its building was in disrepair and there was uncertainty about whether it should be extensively refurbished or whether it should move to a new site in Swanston Street. Morale was low and the finances of the school were in a poor state.

After a meeting with the school and some intense discussions with its senior staff, I decided that we needed to make a fresh start by appointing a new head. After a competitive process, we ended up appointing a non-dentist to the position – a radical step which caused quite a stir amongst the dental profession. Eric Reynolds was a senior scientist in the school, attracting a lot of NHMRC support for his research. He had discovered a peptide which helped to prevent dental caries and could be added to toothpaste. This has since been successfully commercialised. Eric soon earned the confidence of the staff of the school and, in time, that of the wider dental profession. He has proved to be an outstanding head of the school, and importantly, his research has continued to flourish despite the demands of administration. The dental school did move to a new building on Swanston Street, providing it with modern facilities, albeit with inadequate space.

Another interesting challenge during my time as dean was to sort out issues relating to conflict of interest. The head of one of the departments, an internationally renowned expert in the field, was the chief scientific officer of a company set up to develop new therapies based on a discovery he had made. This was all admirable. But a potential conflict of interest emerged as the company was contracting research to the department of which he was head. The university ruled that it was not appropriate for someone who had a significant role in a company which was funding research in a department to be head of that department, because of the possibility of real or perceived conflict of interest. This was an example of the complexities that can come from universities commercialising their research and undertaking contract research for private companies.

Internal allocation of funds within universities is always a controversial and hotly contested topic. The University of Melbourne was no exception. The funding weights for humanities, education and law had been modified from those used in attracting funds to the university in a way which was very advantageous to those disciplines at the expense of medicine, engineering and science. Moreover, substantial funds were taken 'off the top' of the funding for the indirect costs of research by the central university. Some of this was of course justified, but from the perspective of the Faculty of Medicine, Dentistry and Health Sciences, many of the researchers felt that they were disadvantaged compared with the return of infrastructure funds to researchers in other universities.

The annual budget discussions at the university culminated in a three-day retreat for the senior university administration and the deans at Lindenderry, a very nice resort and winery on the Mornington Peninsula. It will forever be etched in my memory for the drama which occurred at these retreats. They were highly theatrical and charged events, at which the pros and cons of different funding models were debated. It was a very testing time for the deans, as decisions that were made could theoretically have major funding implications for their faculty. At my first or second involvement in this process, the vice-chancellor responded to concerns I had expressed by indicating that he wanted a new funding formula to provide more funds to support research with the general principle that since we wished to be a research-intensive university, a higher proportion of the return to faculties should be based on research output. A new formula was concocted which seemed reasonable at face value. When it was modelled using current data, it showed that the Faculty of Medicine, Dentistry and Health Sciences would receive about AUS$8 million per year extra. The other faculties, of course, were not impressed and suggested alterations to the weightings in the formula. The sums were

CHAPTER 14

recalculated overnight and again it showed that there would be an extra AUS$8 million for our faculty. Vice-Chancellor Alan Gilbert, said that this demonstrated the robustness of the concept, as two different formulae had given the same outcome. It was decided that this should be phased in gradually, starting in two years. Of course, before it was implemented, the faculties that were to be disadvantaged persuaded the vice-chancellor to change the formula substantially, so in the end there was only marginal redistribution of funds to encourage research-intensive and expensive faculties.

The perceived disadvantage felt by researchers working within the faculty's schools and departments was exacerbated when the vice-chancellor and deputy vice-chancellor (research), Frank Larkins (no relation), decided to encourage the medical research institutes to have their research grants submitted through the university, which would result in the University of Melbourne increasing its reported research income, an important metric for ranking within Australia and internationally. As an inducement, the university offered to return 85 per cent of the commonwealth's funding for the indirect costs of research to the institutes, a much more favourable return than occurred for the university's own departments. After spirited protest, I managed to have the university agree that 15 per cent of such funds should come to the faculty, which we could use to supplement the indirect costs of researchers within the faculty.

The relationship between universities with medical schools and their affiliated medical research institutes is a complex and troublesome one. At a simple level, the closer the relationship, the better. The medical research institutes contribute much to the advancement of knowledge and to the training of future researchers through the large number of PhD students they have. Their scientists also often contribute to education, usually in a modest way, with lectures and sometimes by undergraduate student research placements. But by and large, the institutes value their independence, they are governed by boards which often include powerful business people, and they are suspicious of the attempts by universities to work more closely with them. It was an unresolved issue while I was dean, although I was an ex officio member of the boards of several of the institutes and attempted to draw them closer to the university because of the scientific and educational benefit which would flow to both through a genuinely collaborative approach driven predominantly by research and education outcomes.

The relationship between university staff and the staff specialists in the major teaching hospitals is also complex. Most of the senior hospital staff are granted university titles of one sort or another. Those up to associate professor are granted by the faculty. Some positions of director of hospital departments are agreed after negotiation with the university to be professor and director appointments and a joint appointment committee made up of nominees of the hospital and the university makes the appointment. The university representatives confer the title. Professorial titles can also be conferred on other hospital staff by a university committee, usually in recognition of outstanding contributions to research.

Shortly after I was appointed as dean, I was called to a meeting with the deputy vice-chancellors Frank Larkins and Boris Schedvin. They said that one of my objectives during my time as dean should be to clarify the distinction between hospital and university appointments. I replied that on the contrary, I hoped that by the time I finished as dean, the distinction between university and hospital staff would be even harder to define and identify. All staff of a teaching hospital, I felt, should feel part of a single enterprise that comprised the highest quality patient care and education at all levels for all health professionals, and research that ranged across the spectrum, covering health services and public health research, clinical and translational research, and basic research focused on areas of clinical relevance. The discussion highlighted one of the many reasons that universities regard their medical faculties as mixed blessings – they wouldn't be without them, but they do cause a lot of headaches.

Suzanne Cory was the director of the Walter and Eliza Hall Institute, an outstanding medical research institute which, under the successive leadership of Sir Macfarlane Burnet, Sir Gustav Nossal and now Suzanne Cory, had established itself as the clear leader in basic medical research in Australia, especially in the fields of immunology and cancer. Before I became dean, while I was still professor of medicine at Royal Melbourne Hospital, Suzanne and I discussed how we could get more collaboration between the medical research institutes and hospitals affiliated with the University of Melbourne. We also recognised the potential for there to be a new facility which would help multidisciplinary research and commercial partnerships. The veterinary precinct immediately adjoining the Royal Melbourne Hospital had a significant

CHAPTER 14

amount of its land becoming available. We convinced the administration of Royal Melbourne Hospital of the benefits of such a partnership.

When I became dean, Suzanne and I brought together the eighteen or so institutes and major teaching hospitals associated with the University of Melbourne under the banner of Bio 21, a reference to the twenty-first century. Fortuitously, we discussed the potential of a new building with Daryl Jackson, the architect who had designed the Walter and Eliza Hall Institute building in the 1980s as well as many other prestigious projects. He referred to an 'anonymous donor' who had made a very major donation to the University of Queensland and who had a particular interest in supporting medical research. It turned out that an old associate of mine, Ron Clarke, the holder of many world records for running in the 1960s, was working for the donor at that time. I knew Clarke through my college roommate, Stanley Spittle, who was also a runner. Daryl Jackson and Ron Clarke arranged a meeting between me, the vice-chancellor, Suzanne Cory and the donor, who turned out to be Chuck Feeney, an Irish-American. Feeney had made a fortune from duty-free stores and was determined to give most of it away. Medical research in Australia was a favourite cause, although up till then and to a large extent since, Queensland was his favoured venue.

We explained our vision for collaboration and the huge potential effectiveness of the partners if they worked collaboratively together. Eventually, Chuck Feeney made a donation of AUS$30 million for the University of Melbourne and AUS$20 million for the Walter and Eliza Hall Institute, with the condition that matching funding had to be obtained. In the case of the university, it had recently had a windfall with the sale of its subsidiary, Melbourne IT, with a return of AUS$85 million to the university. This enabled the university to commit AUS$45 million to a new building, and the state committed transfer of crown land on the veterinary precinct and AUS$16 million cash towards the project. So funds had been obtained for a new building which would become the centrepiece of the new enterprise, the Bio 21 Cluster.

With the state money came constraints about both the structure and role of Bio 21. John Brumby, the state treasurer and minister for innovation, was passionate about the potential of medical research and biotechnology to transform the economy of Victoria and was determined that the state money contributed to the Bio 21 exercise should be used to catalyse commercial returns through the generation of intellectual property, licensing agreements and spin-out companies. The agreement signed by the university (now taken out of my hands) agreed to establish an incorporated company with a commercial board led by a prominent businessman. When I expressed my concerns about the commercial nature of the agreement undermining the Bio 21 concept, I was told not to worry: it was important to satisfy the government's requirements in order to release their money, and everything would be all right.

Roland Williams, the appointed chair of the Bio 21 board, had had a very distinguished career in the resources field and was the president of the Business and Higher Education Round Table. At great expense, an international chief executive officer was hired, a doctor who worked in the pharmaceutical industry. As the great potential of the 'Parkville strip' and beyond was harnessed, huge commercial returns were projected.

I was aghast at these developments, as the Bio 21 concept was about achieving collaboration for the benefits of medical research and ultimately for the benefit of the community. Each of the partners had its own commercialisation program and regarded the intellectual property they generated as belonging to it; they were not prepared to cede it to Bio 21. Indeed, the apparent requirement to do this would guarantee that as soon as any extra funding was exhausted, the cluster would fall apart. The CEO was not equipped to handle this complex situation.

I called a meeting of all the members, which I described as a meeting of the real Bio 21. Doug Daines, who was the director of buildings and facilities and represented the university on the board of the Bio 21 company, suggested I should cancel the meeting, as it would cause confusion. I ignored the suggestion and the meeting went ahead. I again enunciated my conviction that the purpose of Bio 21 was about gaining collaboration, sharing research platforms and achieving more scientific success. Successful commercialisation would be a by-product, but except by prior arrangement, and in exceptional circumstances where the role of Bio 21 in generating the intellectual property was clear, the intellectual property would continue to belong to the institution or institutions where it had been created.

The folly of the commercial structure and focus was then realised. A new structure was established and, under the chairmanship of David Penington, the Bio 21 Cluster became an effective body. It went from strength to strength when my old research colleague, the indomitable Stella Clark, was appointed as CEO. It has achieved a great deal in fostering research

CHAPTER 14

collaboration, shared research platforms, translational research and research in hospitals and it has developed a program of research opportunities for undergraduates (UROP). The Bio 21 Institute is a focus of research activity, particularly in chemistry and biochemistry, and also houses a branch of CSL. The ambitious plan for biotechnology incubators has not taken off, but overall the Bio 21 Cluster has achieved much of what of Suzanne Cory and I originally envisaged despite the false steps along the way.

With the relocation of the dental hospital and the dental school to a new site on Swanston Street, discussions commenced on the possible uses of the old dental hospital site, a triangular block bounded by Grattan Street to the north, Elizabeth Street to the east and Flemington Road to the south-west. As this was immediately across Grattan Street from the Royal Melbourne Hospital and diagonally across Elizabeth Street from the University of Melbourne, it was a very strategic site for future development for a hospital or a medical research institute. Although the state government which owned the land contemplated its sale for a hotel, apartment block or office block development, Minister Brumby was readily persuaded of its potential role in building the medical research capacity of the Parkville strip. There were two main possibilities. It could either be the site of a relocated Peter MacCallum Cancer Centre, or else it could add to the potential of the Bio 21 development by forming a 'research hotel' to provide temporary accommodation for commercial start-up companies or research and development operations of biotechnology companies. Given that there was enough space on the veterinary precinct to the west of the Royal Melbourne Hospital to accommodate the 'research hotel' concept, if there should be a demand for such a facility, it seemed much more strategic to attempt to relocate the Peter MacCallum Cancer Centre (the 'Peter Mac') to the dental hospital site.

This was not as straightforward as it might seem. There was a lot of historical baggage relating to the location of the Peter Mac at its site in East Melbourne. Originally, this specialist cancer hospital had started its life in 1950 as the Victorian centre for radiotherapy treatment for cancer patients located at a central city site in William Street. When this site was felt to be inadequate in the 1980s, there had been considerable public debate and controversy about where the new hospital should be located. By this time, its range of activity had broadened to include all forms of cancer treatment, including chemotherapy and surgery as well as radiotherapy. In some ways, it could be seen as competing with the large general hospitals, such as Royal Melbourne Hospital in the management of patients with cancer. No radiotherapy was available in the general hospitals and patients deemed to require radiotherapy were either transported to the Peter Mac daily to receive the treatment or transferred to the Peter Mac if there were not other causes for continuing treatment in the general hospital. Peter Mac had no emergency department, only a rudimentary intensive care and the availability of the range of non-cancer specialist services that cancer patients often require was limited.

It seemed logical to me and many others that it would be best to collocate the new Peter Mac with a major general hospital, and given the proximity to the Walter and Eliza Hall Institute and the University of Melbourne, the Royal Melbourne site seemed the most appropriate. We lobbied hard for this outcome, but the Peter Mac was opposed to it because its board and staff believed that it would lose its autonomy and that its ability to provide outstanding care to patients with cancer would be jeopardised. There was no doubt that the Peter Mac did provide outstanding pastoral care and support for its patients and high quality cancer treatment. The controversy was very public and I and others, including David Penington, campaigned actively for what we felt would be the best long-term outcome: Peter Mac collocated with the Royal Melbourne.

The premier at the time, John Cain, was sympathetic to the wish of Peter Mac to stay geographically separate from the Royal Melbourne. The decision was taken to relocate the Peter Mac to East Melbourne, where a private hospital, St Andrews, had become non-viable and available for purchase. So in 1988, the Peter Mac moved to East Melbourne. The site was modified and clinical and research facilities enlarged. However, by 2000 it was apparent that the current facility was inadequate in size and inappropriate in structure to support the increased demand for cancer services and the very impressive research activities in the hospital. So discussions commenced between the Peter Mac (with its board chaired by Heather Wellington), the Royal Melbourne Hospital (with its board chaired by David Karpin) and the university, represented by me as the dean. The same wariness of the Peter Mac about the possibility of losing its autonomy and being taken over by the Royal Melbourne surfaced again. The state government called for a report by consultants. Although the consultants' report was supportive of relocation, the relations between the Peter Mac and Royal Melbourne were

CHAPTER 14

still tense and the state government was not at that time in a position to raise the estimated AUS$400 million required for the relocation.

As a postscript to these discussions, it is gratifying that by 2009 the state and commonwealth governments had agreed to provide the bulk of the funding to allow a AUS$1.1 billion development that would include the relocation of the Peter Mac to the dental hospital site, three new stories for cancer treatment at the Royal Melbourne Hospital connected to the new Peter Mac by walkways over Grattan Street and new research facilities for the University of Melbourne. In addition to the new facilities, a functional consortium known as the Victorian Comprehensive Cancer Centre was formed to bring together the cancer services, cancer education and the cancer research of the Peter Mac, Melbourne Health (Royal Melbourne Hospital), the Royal Women's Hospital, the Royal Children's Hospital, the University of Melbourne, the Walter and Eliza Hall Institute and the more remotely located Western Hospital and St Vincent's Hospital under a joint venture structure. Ironically, I was asked by the health minister of the Brumby state government, Daniel Andrews, to chair the joint venture board, and this has continued under Minister David Davis of the coalition Baillieu-Napthine governments. Recently, the Murdoch Children's Research Institute and the Austin Hospital have joined the consortium.

As with most schools of medicine in Australia at that time, international engagement was a major priority. Of course, there were financial incentives for this, with the budget of the faculty being very dependent on the income from international students who paid fees which were realistic in terms of the cost of delivery of the course, unlike the heavily subsidised fees we were able to charge Australian students. The students came from many countries, with South-East Asia the dominant region from which the medical and dental schools attracted students (and Malaysia and Singapore the most represented nations of that region). As well as the financial benefit, the faculty saw great advantage in the diversity brought to the faculty by these students and attempted to broaden the source countries, particularly by developing a relationship with the University of Botswana, not only taking students from that country, but also helping the university in its plans to develop a medical school of its own. Getting to know the highly engaging academics from the University of Botswana, the politicians and bureaucrats and then visiting the university and the main hospital (Princess Marina) in Gaborone was one highlight of my time as dean. Their positive attitude, despite the devastating impact of the HIV-AIDS epidemic, was inspiring, and unlike some of the South African leaders, the politicians and bureaucrats in Botswana were taking enlightened and positive steps in the prevention of spread and the treatment of those infected.

I was invited to speak at a symposium to celebrate the ninetieth anniversary of the Peking University Health Science Centre. Until then, it had been independent of Beijing (Peking) University, but as was occurring elsewhere in China, its days as a separate university were rapidly drawing to a close and it was soon to be amalgamated with Beijing University. At that visit, I was assigned a bright young nursing student as a guide and interpreter. She was keen to learn as much as she could about the West. In a highly orchestrated student concert in which the glories of China and its leaders were the subject of almost every highly patriotic song and dance, the student, after translating the words of one of the songs, asked me quietly whether students in Australia would sing songs like this. I was forced to concede that they would not.

The student exemplified the entrepreneurial spirit necessary for success in the highly competitive environment of China. She really wanted to do medicine, not nursing, but had been assigned to nursing. Somehow, she managed to gain a place in biomedical science at the State University of New York and from there gained entry to medicine. She had maintained email contact with me till that point and I had acted as a referee to the extent that I could. She has now completed her medical degree and is a surgical trainee.

In a visit to Malaysia for alumni events and hospital visits, it was a little galling to hear from Malaysian medical alumni that they wondered what the University of Melbourne was doing, as Monash University was so much more prominent there, partly because of the campus that university had established at Sunway. Even though the Sunway campus of Monash did not at that stage have a medical school, the profile of the whole university had been raised by the presence of the campus.

The role of a dean of a compound faculty of medicine and health sciences is a complex one. Not only is there all the internal university politics entailing the somewhat ambiguous role of trying to act in the best interests of your faculty while being a good and collegial corporate citizen trying to act in the interests of the university as a whole, but there is also the need to manage the often conflicting interests between the different schools and departments

CHAPTER 14

within the faculty. More broadly, there is a need to interact at the state and commonwealth levels with the health bureaucracies and politicians.

The university-wide role was a particularly interesting one. The vice-chancellor, Alan Gilbert, a man of great intelligence and charm, was a visionary whose vision was sometimes a little beyond that of his senior management and indeed ahead of its time.

There were two major university-wide initiatives during his time as vice-chancellor.

The first was the creation of Melbourne University Private. The rationale was that the public universities were struggling under the constraints of government regulation and their own cumbersome processes that meant they were unable to deliver flexible offerings meeting the needs of students and particularly the corporate sector. After attempting to get private co-investment, the university borrowed money and embarked on an ambitious building program to create the private university in University Square, immediately across Grattan Street to the south of the existing university campus. Permission was granted by the state government to establish the university, although there were constraints, including the need to demonstrate research activity. Initial areas contemplated were in business, communications and the environment with custom-built masters programs for corporate clients. Alan presented his plans at the annual heads and deans retreat at Lorne and asked for comments. I was the only one silly enough to comment. I said that although his presentation was compelling and inspirational, I thought there were some fundamental flaws in the plan. The first was that he was aiming at the graduate market. Graduate and postgraduate education was already largely deregulated in the public sector – any courses could be created, any number of students admitted and the fees charged were at the discretion of the university. Moreover, the university already had the Melbourne Business School operating as a controlled entity able to do anything in the business area that Melbourne University Private could do, and the course offerings would be in potential competition with the graduate courses offered by the faculties of the public university. It was planned that staff could teach in both the private and public universities, but again the financial attractions of the private university might well be against the interests of the public university.

There were a number of iterations of the academic plans for the private university. It never achieved a critical mass of students and ultimately was closed by Glyn Davis when he became vice-chancellor of the University of

Melbourne in 2004. Although the private university did not succeed, the ambitious building program the vision engendered has been of great benefit to the university and will be a lasting legacy to Alan Gilbert.

The second visionary idea was to create an international network of universities of like type around the world. Some of the universities involved in U21 were University of Queensland and University of New South Wales in Australia, Auckland University, the National University of Singapore, Hong Kong University, Fudan University in Shanghai, the universities of Nottingham, Birmingham, Glasgow and Edinburgh in the United Kingdom, and the University of British Columbia in Canada. The number and membership have changed from time to time, but this core remains.

U21 had two major objectives. One was to achieve a basis for collaborative forums for the university administrations and for the academic staff in the different disciplines so that they could share knowledge and resources in education, research and policy. From the point of view of my own discipline, medicine and health sciences, it provided a helpful and constructive forum, with an initial meeting in Singapore in 2000 and essentially annual meetings since then. Apart from getting to know colleagues around the world who were wrestling with the same problems, the forum was a great help in sharing policies relating, for example, to students with disabilities and to the sharing of best practice with respect to new teaching methodologies. An initiative to set up a shared repository of educational resources was too ambitious – there were problems with intellectual property, rapid obsolescence of electronic resources and the ready availability of such resources for open access via the internet.

U21 has also offered staff and student exchange scholarships and fellowships. Overall, although all the objectives of the U21 partnership have not been realised, significant benefits have flowed to the participant universities and certainly did to our faculty.

The other objective of U21 has not been so successful. The plan was to form U21 Global in partnership with an international media or educational network to deliver U21-badged university courses by the internet to the vast potential market of students wishing to gain a quality university degree with little chance of travelling and gaining admission to an elite university. Alan Gilbert took leave of absence from the university for six months and left the newly appointed senior deputy vice-chancellor Sally Walker in charge while Alan went to the UK to negotiate, initially with News Limited and

CHAPTER 14

later with Thomson Learning, to achieve a commercial partner. Thomson Learning, a large international company headquartered in Canada, became the commercial partner.

Despite a large amount of effort by many people, the cyber version of U21 did not take off. There were a number of reasons for this. First, it was difficult to get the same enthusiasm from the other universities and their staff to contribute their time and intellectual property to the initiative. Second, there were already providers of online university education that had much more experience in the logistics of such an operation. Third, it was hard to get much student enthusiasm to embark on expensive online degree courses that were badged not by a well-known university itself, but by the somewhat elusive concept of a consortium of universities with the poorly recognised and somewhat ambiguous name of U21 Global (was it twenty-one universities or the twenty-first century?).

One can imagine that it was a tumultuous time at the University of Melbourne. The dual initiatives of Melbourne University Private and U21 Global occupied a lot of time and engendered fierce debate at the professorial board. Although neither project succeeded in the way that Alan imagined they might, they certainly shook the university out of any complacency that might have embraced it and led to a lot of side benefits for the university.

The international relations which were enhanced by these initiatives, together with international activities of the College of Physicians, had other benefits. In 2001, I was contacted by an old friend and colleague, Professor Tan Chorh Chuan, to take part in a committee to review life sciences education in Singapore. Professor Tan had been seconded from his definitive position of the dean of medicine at the National University of Singapore to be the director of clinical services for the Ministry of Health in Singapore. He was later appointed vice-chancellor and president of NUS.

The committee was to be chaired by Lord Ron Oxburgh, recently retired as the rector of Imperial College, and comprised the dean of medicine from Johns Hopkins in Baltimore, the professor of medicine from Oxford, the dean of medicine from the Lund University as well as me. It was to report directly to deputy prime minister of Singapore, Tony Tan. The motivation to establish this committee had come from the chair of the Economic Development Board of Singapore, the dynamic Philip Yeo. The EDB had decided that life sciences research and the industry surrounding it should be the next plank in the economic development of Singapore.

As is often the case, the review was immensely valuable for those taking part. We shared views and experiences with each other. We also had an opportunity to examine at first hand the single-minded and strategic approach which Singapore was taking to its economic development. The lack of a significant electoral threat to the incumbent government meant that it could take a long-term strategic view rather than concentrating on short-term populist policies, which are encouraged by our three-year, hotly contested electoral cycle.

The decision that life sciences was to be the next major plank in economic development had been accompanied by a number of initiatives to support this. These included major financial inducements to pharmaceutical companies to set up Asia Pacific headquarters in Singapore, a huge financial commitment to develop a new hub for life sciences research (Biopolis), bringing together university researchers, medical research institute researchers and industry. It also had a strategy for attracting high quality and prestigious international researchers to Singapore, either as definitive appointments or for substantial periods each year. Together, billions of dollars had been committed to these strategies.

An identified problem that our panel was meant to address was how to reform medical education to encourage more graduates to undertake research, as a lack of home-grown clinician scientists was seen as a major shortcoming. There was also a proposal to establish a second medical school, perhaps at the Nanyang Technical University, to provide more doctors and competition for the NUS medical school. This was being pushed by the Singapore General Hospital, which felt that it had been marginalised in terms of medical education following the construction of the National University Hospital.

After a number of meetings in Singapore and London, the panel made many recommendations. It did not think that Nanyang Technical University had sufficient expertise in life sciences and medical humanities to support a medical school at that stage, but that there was a strong argument for a graduate-entry medical program based around the Singapore General Hospital. This could be a second program for NUS or done in company with another medical school outside Singapore.

In response to the report, a graduate-entry medical school was established based around SGH, initially involving a partnership between that hospital, NUS and Duke University in the USA. Several years later, a medical school was started at Nanyang Technical University.

CHAPTER 14

The overwhelming message for me from the review was the need for Australia or one or more of its states to make a strategic long-term commitment to life sciences research if we were to remain internationally competitive. There have certainly been instances of this mainly driven by individual states, but also with the commonwealth increasing the funding of NHMRC. Moreover, our medical education system and historical precedents are much more supportive of high quality medical graduates being attracted to research working in association with science graduates. Singapore is making remarkable progress, but changing a culture to achieve the ends they wish is not simple. For this reason, Australia has remained competitive in medical research, although this is not assured into the future.

Alan Gilbert was fiercely ambitious for the reputation of the University of Melbourne. A method of ranking the world's universities on the basis of their research performance devised by the Shanghai Jiaotong University had emerged. As well as research publications and citations and other crude indicators of research standing, the number of alumni and staff members who had received Nobel Prizes (or the mathematical equivalent, the Fields Medal) was accorded significant weight in the ranking system. In a characteristically proactive way, the vice-chancellor offered a financial incentive of AUS$100,000 per year to any faculty able to attract a Nobel Prize winner to the staff for a period of greater than two months per year for three years.

I regarded the initiative as a bit cynical, so did not think that our faculty would actively pursue the reward unless it happened fortuitously. We constantly sought through our schools and departments to recruit high quality research staff who would help our research effort, regardless of whether or not they had won a Nobel Prize.

By coincidence, Caroline and I were invited to have dinner by a neurosurgical colleague, David Wallace, who was entertaining a German scientist and his wife, who were visiting Melbourne to attend the Australian Tennis Open. The neurosurgeon's son was a scientist who had visited the Max Planck Institute in Heidelberg, directed by the scientist. It turned out that the scientist was the neurophysiologist Bert Sakmann, who had been awarded the Nobel Prize jointly with Erwin Neher in 1991 for his discovery of the patch clamp technique and the identification and elucidation of the role of ion channels in the activation of nerve cells. We were not able to accept the invitation to dinner, but did follow up by contacting Bert Sakmann and inviting him to come to work in the faculty for two months over the next three years. Being very positive about his visit to Australia, he accepted.

On his first visit, the vice-chancellor was keen to generate as much publicity as possible for the university based on its success in attracting a German Nobel Laureate to come and work at the university. Meanwhile, Bert was busy establishing scientific collaborations and quickly became enthused about the quality of the neuroscience that was being performed at the university and particularly about the opportunities to extend his research on ion channels to identifying the role of a gene identified by neuroscientists in the Austin Hospital department of medicine as the cause of an uncommon form of familial epilepsy. It was a fruitful collaboration of a type not possible at the Max Planck, which had relatively poorly developed links with clinical researchers. He valued particularly the degree of scientific training and dedication to research he found in many Australian clinicians and felt he could do clinically relevant research in Melbourne that was impossible in Germany.

On his next visit, Bert asked me to keep the visit secret so that he could concentrate on the science rather than being paraded as a prize exhibit.

While in Melbourne, Bert and his wife, Christianne, were offered accommodation in Trinity College. They greatly enjoyed participation in the life of the college and in interacting with the students. Bert was, however, a bit perturbed when he was asked to read a lesson in the chapel. Trinity was holding an arts festival, celebrating the creativity of its students. The lesson chosen for Bert was designed to celebrate the general theme of creativity, so he was asked to read the first chapter of Genesis describing the Creation. Bert felt that he might be being set up by creationists, but I was able to reassure him that Trinity College was not a stronghold of those who believed literally in the story of Creation and that there was no ulterior motive behind his being asked to read this chapter. I hoped I was right. In any case, he dutifully read the chapter without adverse outcomes or publicity.

Bert Sakmann was an inspirational figure for the young neuroscientists working in the university and in the Howard Florey Institute. In turn, he enjoyed his visits very much and felt he could do research there that he could not undertake elsewhere. He continued to visit after his original contractual arrangement had finished.

We managed to attract another Nobel Prize winner to the university. Peter Doherty was an Australian who had been awarded the Nobel Prize

CHAPTER 14

for Physiology or Medicine jointly with a Swiss, Rolf Zinkernagel, for work performed at the Australian National University in the 1970s. They had demonstrated that alterations to the HLA antigens on the surface of cells infected with virus allowed the body's killer T cells to recognise the infected cells and attempt to eliminate them. Doherty had been working for a number of years at St Jude's Hospital for Children in Memphis. He was quite keen to return to Australia but was anxious to have the right circumstances to support his research and to allow continuing collaboration with his co-workers at St Jude's. After detailed and protracted negotiations, we were able to persuade Peter to return to Australia with his wife, Penny. Peter was given a laboratory in the microbiology department and worked in Australia for nine months and spent approximately three months each year in Memphis.

As in the case of Bert Sakmann, this was a very successful appointment, and Peter continues to undertake research and mentor young scientists at the university.

So despite my scepticism, Alan Gilbert's scheme for attracting Nobel Prize winners worked out very well for the faculty.

Chapter 15

CHAIR OF THE NATIONAL HEALTH AND MEDICAL RESEARCH COUNCIL

The National Health and Medical Research Council (NHMRC) was established in the 1930s to advise the government on matters relating to health and to develop a strategy and administer funding for health and medical research. A function relating to health ethics was added later. It now has three principal committees, the Research Committee, the Health Advisory Committee and the Australian Health Ethics Committee. The chairs of NHMRC and its principal committees are appointed by the commonwealth government on the advice of the minister for health. Although it was administered through the department of health, the chair has a direct reporting line to the minister.

In February 1997, I received a phone call from my long-time colleague and friend, Richard Smallwood, who had been chair of NHMRC from 1995 to 1997. He said that I would be receiving a phone call from the minister for health, Dr Michael Wooldridge, inviting me to become chair of NHMRC. He went on to advise me that I should not accept, as it was a poisoned chalice.

This came out of the blue, as I had no expectation or ambition to be chair of NHMRC. Indeed, another colleague and friend, John Funder, had mentioned to me that the minister was nominating him for the position. Smallwood explained to me that the independent, Senator Brian Harradine, who held the balance of power in the Senate had questioned the appointment of Funder. Senator Harradine was a passionate advocate for the interests of his home state, Tasmania, but was also a staunch Roman Catholic and fiercely opposed to abortion. At that time, there was a controversy about the approval by the government of the use of the 'abortion drug' RU 486

CHAPTER 15

in Australia. Apparently, John Funder had advocated its use, although this had been done in a scientific context. Although Harradine later denied that this was the basis for his questioning Funder's appointment, this was the commonly perceived interpretation. For whatever reason, Smallwood said that Funder, despite his impeccable scientific credentials and a high and worthy public and academic profile, would not get Harradine's support for appointment as chair of NHMRC and moreover that if that appointment went ahead, there was a fear that he would block other legislation felt important by the Liberal coalition (conservative) government.

As I was vice-president of the Royal Australasian College of Physicians at the time, with a reasonable expectation of becoming president in 1998, and likely to succeed Gordon Clunie as the dean of the Faculty of Medicine, Dentistry and Health Sciences at the beginning of 1998, I was very comfortable with Richard Smallwood's advice. This feeling was reinforced by my opposition to the form of political interference in what I felt to be the totally appropriate appointment of John Funder as chair of NHMRC. Moreover, I shared his support for the abortion drug RU 486.

I was therefore surprised to receive another call from Richard Smallwood the next evening telling me that the call from the minister was still going to come but reversing his earlier advice. He said that I had to take the position when it was offered, as the future of medical research funding was dependent on the minister finding a way out of the impasse with Senator Harradine. If he failed to do this, the forward commitment of funding for medical research was likely to be threatened.

Sure enough, two days later, I received the phone call from Michael Wooldridge asking me to come to his electorate office in Box Hill the next day (Sunday), as he had an important matter to discuss with me. I had only met Dr Wooldridge once before at a dinner, where he had spoken. We had had a brief but heated disagreement about the number of doctors being trained. He expressed the opinion that there were too many and I disagreed. He either did not recall this or chose not to refer to it.

He raised the issue of the chair of NHMRC and briefed me about the difficulty that he had encountered. He emphasised that the future funding of medical research through NHMRC was perilous, as although there had been some recent increases, these had not been built into the forward estimates by the Treasury. This meant that in three years or so, the level of NHMRC funding would fall back to that before the increase. Since grants and fellowships are usually allocated on a three to five-year basis, the forward commitments following the recent increase in funding would take up nearly all the available funds. This would mean that no or very few grants and fellowships could be awarded, with catastrophic consequences for the whole health and medical research community. Many researchers would lose their jobs, with outstanding people likely to be lost to the research sector forever. This was a persuasive argument. I asked for time to consider whether I would accept such a position. Interestingly, I was not asked my views on RU 486 or on abortion.

The situation was complicated by the media publicity at the time. A number of my medical colleagues had been quoted publicly deploring the political interference with the appointment and supporting John Funder. Accepting the position would seem like a betrayal of the principle of an independent NHMRC.

I spent the next couple of days phoning many colleagues in medical research, including a direct conversation with John Funder. I was advised by everyone, including John, that I should take the position and indeed that it was important that I do so.

I therefore phoned Michael Wooldridge and indicated that I was prepared to accept the position. There was a further media flurry, which included a photograph of me on the front page of the *Australian* taken with the shadows of some bars on a window over my face, making it look as if I was imprisoned. I was also interviewed for the *7.30 Report* by a charming young woman, with whom I had a relaxed and informal conversation before the cameras rolled. Once the cameras were started, she moved straight to the point and asked, 'Well, Professor Larkins, how does it feel to be second choice?'

And I had thought that she was my friend. I battled through the interview and when it concluded she said, 'You win'. The interview was not screened, which I took as a minor triumph.

Although the media interest rapidly subsided and the medical research community was supportive of my appointment, it was the beginning of a difficult six months. Michael Wooldridge was not in a rush to complete the process of appointing the council of NHMRC, although he did appoint chairs of the principal committees. Professor Stephen Leeder, a highly respected professor of public health at the University of Sydney was appointed as chair of the Health Advisory Committee, Professor Warwick Anderson, the professor of physiology at Monash University was appointed

CHAPTER 15

as chair of the Research Committee, Don Chalmers was appointed as chair of the Australian Health Ethics Committee and Dr Jack Best, a health consultant with previous experience in many different areas, including medical research, public health, rural health strategy, health economics and workforce, was appointed as the chair of a new principal committee styled the Strategic Research Advisory Committee. The council was embedded in the department of health, with its CEO being effectively a deputy secretary of the department, Dallas Ariotti, a very capable individual, who we were soon to discover had a fiery disposition.

The first meeting of the executive was called shortly after the appointment of the chairs of the principal committees and some months before the rest of the council was finally appointed. It was clear that Dallas was tense because of all the political heat around the NHMRC and an impending Senate Estimates hearing. Stephen Leeder, in his inimitable fashion, started to expound on his views of the NHMRC, public health policy and the world in general. Before we knew it, Dallas had stormed out of our first meeting and announced her resignation as the CEO of NHMRC. Hardly an auspicious start. Dallas subsequently moved to the UK with her husband, Professor William Doe, who was appointed as the dean of the medical school at the University of Birmingham. She has had a distinguished career in the health service in the UK, demonstrating great leadership during the station and bus bombings of 2005.

Warwick and I came up with suggestions for membership of the Research Committee, but Minister Wooldridge was a little 'gun-shy' and said that he was reluctant to appoint people to it, or to the council itself, whom he didn't know personally. Eventually, some months into the new triennium, the appointments were made.

The council in those days was a large and cumbersome beast with around thirty-two members. As well as the chief executives of health, or occasionally their nominees from each of the states and territories, the chief medical officer of the commonwealth, other commonwealth officials and the chairs of the principal committees, there were a number of ministerial appointments (approved by cabinet). These included Margaret Guilfoyle, the minister for finance in the Fraser government, and a young student, Celia Kemp, who was in the fourth year of a combined medicine and law degree and the niece of a senior commonwealth minister, David Kemp, then minister for education. I was concerned by what could be perceived as the political nature of these appointments, but both turned out to be excellent and unbiased members of the council, whose input I valued enormously. There were also nominees from the Aboriginal and Torres Strait Islander Council (ATSIC, since disbanded) and individuals nominated for their experience and expertise as consumer representatives.

The new NHMRC was required to present its strategic plan for the next triennium to parliament within about three weeks of its formation. Given the controversy around its chair and membership and the lack of time for a collegial atmosphere to be built amongst the council members, this was a tall order. There was no time for the type of consultation process that one would like to follow in formulating this type of document. I felt that the only way we could achieve the objective was to prepare a draft to discuss. Following meetings of our executive, I drew up a draft for discussion by the new council. It was a major topic for discussion in our first council meeting held shortly after in Hobart. After intensive discussion and valuable input from the council, it was agreed and presented to the minister in the required time frame.

After the early days, the members of the council gradually developed confidence in each other and we really felt we started to make significant progress. Much of the action occurred at the level of the principal committees. The Research Committee was landed almost at once with an administrative disaster, Grantnet. Before systems were mature enough and while the internet was still delivering inadequate bandwidth to cope with peak periods of demand, the office of NHMRC had attempted to have online submission of grant applications delivered directly via the internet in real time. The ensuing shambles set the process of handling the annual grants round back substantially. Valuable lessons were learnt at high cost.

The Research Committee embarked on some ambitious reforms, including phasing out block grants to the six large medical research institutes then receiving them. The rationale for this was that it would be fairer to have all the research groups in universities and medical research institutes competing for funds on the same footing, with program grants allowing relatively high funding to be available to productive and innovative groups for five years at a time, the same period as the funding allocation for the institute block grants. Some institutes opposed this quite strongly, with the valid objection that this method of funding prevented the institute senior management and board being able to have discretionary funds to develop new, more

CHAPTER 15

speculative, areas of research or to have the same degree of control over the whole scientific direction of the institute. There are clearly valid arguments on both sides, but I do not think that the subsequent history has indicated that well-performing institutes which were previously block-funded have fared less well, either in a total funding sense or in a strategic sense, than they did under the old system.

The Health Advisory Committee continued to have a valuable role in developing or endorsing evidence-based guidelines in many areas of importance to health care. One of the strategic directions defined in the strategic plan for the triennium had been for NHMRC to work in partnership with other bodies. This was particularly evident in the process of guideline development and endorsement, where a number of other organisations worked with NHMRC in developing guidelines following protocols developed by NHMRC and with NHMRC nominees on the panels. Valuable partnerships with organisations such as the National Heart Foundation, the Australian Diabetes Society, and several others were forged during this time, and increasingly this has become the modus operandi for NHMRC in its health advisory role.

A significant position paper that was discussed at length at the council was that related to the effects of passive smoking on health. Despite threats of legal action from the tobacco industry, an important and influential document was produced.

I was, perhaps naively, disappointed that whenever the minister was interested in a particular area of health care, he established a process outside the department and NHMRC to provide advice. Examples included the Ministerial Advisory Council on Diabetes and a process set up to establish frameworks for introduction of evidence-based care into clinical practice. The latter resulted in formation of a new company, owned by the commonwealth and with the key appointments to its board made by the minister. The National Institute for Clinical Studies did some excellent work but would have been much stronger if it had been incorporated from its inception into the structure of the NHMRC, preferably under the oversight of the Health Advisory Committee. It is clearly an intrinsic characteristic of democracies functioning under the Westminster system for ministers to be reluctant to delegate to committees, once removed from their direct control. Given the flack they receive from the media when things go wrong, it is understandable, but I did find it frustrating.

A major preoccupation for NHMRC shortly after the council was constituted was the Wills Review. The minister for health, Dr Michael Wooldridge, had suggested to Prime Minister Howard that a review of medical research funding, including the National Health and Medical Research Council, was required. The chair of the Garvan Institute, Mr Peter Wills, a prominent Sydney businessman, well-known and respected by John Howard, was chosen to chair the review. His committee comprised in part some prominent researchers, ironically including John Funder. The report that they ultimately published was very influential. Amongst many other recommendations, it advocated a doubling of medical research funding and a new fund of AUS$50 million to fund public health research which it felt could be obtained by pooling funds already spent by state health departments and the commonwealth. The money could, it was felt, be spent more effectively by a peer-review process overseen by NHMRC. The Wills Review also recommended greater separation of the NHMRC from the department of health and greater separation between management and governance of NHMRC. As it was currently operating, the various committees of the council basically ran the research, health advisory and ethics functions of the council with the department of health providing administrative support.

The Wills Review has had a major impact on medical research in Australia. Medical research funding was indeed doubled over the succeeding five years. A chief executive officer of NHMRC was appointed, who took over many of the functions of the chairs of the Research and Health Advisory Committees.

The recommendation for the pool of AUS$50 million to support public health research met a less successful fate. The commonwealth announced at an Australian Health Ministers Advisory Committee meeting that the minister had committed AUS$15 million towards this fund, provided that the states matched it. The representatives of the states said that before putting their money on the table they wanted to know how the money would be dispensed and what it would be used for. The commonwealth replied that once the money was on the table those details could be sorted out. The discussions foundered at that point and nothing came of it.

Dr Jack Best was chair of the newly formed Strategic Research Advisory Committee (SRAC). This was a strange beast, as it would reasonably be expected that the Research Committee would be strategic and not require

CHAPTER 15

the advice of a separate committee. I am not sure that SRAC provided a great deal of strategic advice to the Research Committee, but the inimitable Jack Best was highly innovative in other activities. Notably, he sought to raise awareness of achievement in health and medical research. He inaugurated the 'Tall Poppies' awards for high-achieving, young life scientists, the Florey Medal in recognition of high achievement at the very highest levels of Australian health and medical research and used the centenary of the birth of Australian health and medical researchers of note as a way of raising awareness in young people and the community in general of the importance of medical research and the contributions of Australians.

This started with a number of events to celebrate the contributions of Macfarlane Burnet and continued with Florey and Eccles.

The centenary of the birth of Sir Howard Florey was a particularly notable experience for me. Given that Florey's major research work leading to the development of penicillin occurred at Oxford University during the Second World War, Jack planned a major extravaganza in Oxford to celebrate the event.

The flight over was an experience in its own right. Although I was told I was eligible for a business class fare, I felt that since NHMRC had a limited budget and the purpose of the visit to the UK was not exactly core to the NHMRC mission, I should travel economy. I was rewarded by being next to an extremely obese woman, who was very chatty. She told me that she was going to the UK to see her fiancé in person. She had met him on the Internet. She told me not to worry about her breathing when she slept, as she had sleep apnoea. She had to be taken to a spare seat at the back of the plane to eat her meals, as the tray would not come down over her abdomen. When she left for her meal, she said cheerily to me, 'Don't youse worry. I will be back'. And she did come back. I did not think virtue had been rewarded.

Among other events during the visit, Jack Best arranged a formal dinner at Magdalen College, Oxford hosted by the president of the college, Professor Tony Smith. As chair of NHMRC, I delivered an after-dinner speech on Florey. It was indeed a fine occasion, with the then Australian high commissioner to the UK, Philip Flood, also speaking, and members of the Florey family and Norman Heatley, a member of Florey's team, in attendance.

Heatley was well into his eighties at that time. He was a fine man, not at all bitter about not being included in the Nobel Prize awarded to Florey, Fleming and Chain for the discovery and production of penicillin. His role was vital, as he devised an ingenious method to get large-scale growth of the penicillin mould, a critical step in the production of pharmaceutical quantities of penicillin. He was also involved in most other steps in the process.

My position as chair of NHMRC carried with it membership of some other committees. These included the Prime Minister's Science, Engineering and Innovation Council (PMSEIC), the Australian Health Minister's Advisory Council (AHMAC) and the National Aboriginal and Torres Strait Islander Health Council (NATSIHC).

PMSEIC was an important committee, because it was chaired by the prime minister and was attended by a number of the senior government ministers, although disappointingly, not the treasurer. The meetings were held in the heady atmosphere of the cabinet room of Parliament House. Agendas were arranged by the chief scientist, at that stage, Robin Batterham, and the ministers used the council both as a sounding-board for some new policy initiatives and as a forum to discuss and debate some of the big challenges in science and technology. The non-ministerial members of the council were partly the heads of peak scientific and technical organisations and partly a number of independent members chosen by the prime minister. It was clear that the prime minister, John Howard, treated the council seriously and acted on a number of the recommendations coming from it. Climate change, water policy, the wine industry and funding of health research were amongst many topics discussed.

Together with Hugh Niall and Geoff Brook, I gave a presentation on the potential of the biotechnology sector in Australia, including a discussion of the opportunities and pitfalls in the commercialisation of medical research. Hugh Niall was an outstanding medical researcher, who had then had a distinguished career in the biotechnology industry in the USA and had returned to Australia as the CEO of the Australian biotechnology company Biota, and Geoff Brook was a medical graduate working in a venture capital company in Australia. Together, I think we gave a balanced view, which has been borne out by the subsequent history of biotechnology in this country. Although the actions of the government did not always show it, as members of the council, we felt we were being listened to. I am sure that having this forum to present the findings of the Wills Review was very influential in

CHAPTER 15

the decision by the government to follow the recommendation to double the funding for health and medical research.

It was interesting to return to PMSEIC a decade later as chair of Universities Australia and to see it functioning under the chairmanship of Kevin Rudd. He was also very engaged and took great pleasure in showing that he had both followed the presentations and grasped their essential points by summarising them at the end.

AHMAC was a less edifying experience. It is the forum where the senior commonwealth and state health bureaucrats get together to sort out issues in health policy and funding. As had been highlighted a few years before in Jenny Macklin's report on the National Health Strategy for the Hawke and Keating government, many of the problems in our health care system are related to the divisions of responsibilities for funding and policy between the commonwealth and the states leading to discontinuities of care, cost shifting and inefficiencies. The six monthly meetings of AHMAC should be the forum where these issues are addressed. I was therefore surprised that at the first meeting, one of the state delegates started by saying that there didn't seem to be much on the agenda, so he had changed his flight from the evening to lunchtime. The next forty minutes was taken up with an argument between the representatives of two states about AUS$4000 that one felt that the other owed to the AHMAC budget. At that time, the public budget for health care was about AUS$40 billion, so the $4000 hardly seemed worth the forty-minute debate.

There was a period of intense negotiation every five years in the lead-up to the Australian Health Care Agreement. This was the funding agreement between the commonwealth and the states, by which money was provided by the commonwealth to the states in return for the provision of a range of services, mostly related to running hospitals. Along with the commonwealth chief medical officer, Professor Judith Whitworth and the chair of the Research Committee, Warwick Anderson, we managed to have included in the agreement that in exchange for the commonwealth funding, the states agreed to provide support for research and education in their hospitals. Clearly, this was a loose statement, so AHMAC, at my request, set up a working party to define what was meant and the key performance indicators that might be put in place to ensure that the states were meeting their obligations. Unsurprisingly, there was not a lot of action in this working party. At successive meetings of AHMAC, I would ask of its progress and be told that it was still deliberating. When I finished my term, it still had not concluded this work, and when the tiresome Larkins had departed AHMAC, I think that in the best tradition of the public service, it just stopped meeting.

Notwithstanding the failure to achieve any precision in what it meant, the clause in the 1998 agreement was helpful to those who knew about it. It was used to support the argument that teaching and research were real obligations of the state hospitals and that the hospitals did not solely exist for direct patient care. It has remained a fraught issue – when times are tough, more pressure is put on universities and professional colleges to pay with money they don't have for resources for undergraduate and postgraduate education and research, despite it being in everyone's long-term interests for these to proceed. Attempts to unbundle the costs of medical education and research from the concurrent costs of clinical care delivery are doomed to failure, as confirmed by a government-commissioned study by KPMG.

Clinical medical education and postgraduate training are interwoven with clinical care and clinical research and with clinical outcome evaluation and continuous quality improvement. Consider a typical teaching ward round in a hospital. Information relating to clinical care and education are passed continuously up and down the chain from student-intern to intern to registrar to consultant. The consultant benefits from the new information provided by the registrar and the patient from the more prolonged and fastidious history taken by the student intern, often including aspects of social history ignored by others. As KPMG found, most activities in teaching hospitals are multipurpose and multiproduct, and it is destructive to try to cost them separately.

Chapter 16

THE NATIONAL ABORIGINAL AND TORRES STRAIT ISLANDER HEALTH COUNCIL AND INDIGENOUS HEALTH

The National Aboriginal and Torres Strait Islander Health Council was a new structure formed by Michael Wooldridge to define a strategy for Indigenous health trying to address the dreadful health outcomes in Indigenous communities. Some indicators, such as maternal and neonatal mortality, had improved substantially (although still significantly worse than for the white community) but diabetes, cardiovascular disease and renal disease were having a terrible impact on health status and life expectancy in Indigenous communities. Added to these were a higher incidence of alcohol and other drug problems and mental health issues associated with cultural disruption, unemployment and imprisonment. Living conditions in many remote communities were dreadful, but poor health outcomes affected urbanised as well as remote Indigenous communities.

It was an interesting and challenging committee. It was chaired by the secretary of the department of health, an outstanding public servant called Andrew Podger. I was the only other non-Indigenous member of the committee, although staff of the Office of Aboriginal and Torres Strait Islander Health serviced the council and were in attendance. The other members of the council were Indigenous leaders of health organisations or other notable Indigenous members chosen by the minister for their individual expertise.

The council did not start well. On the first morning, every time Andrew Podger opened his mouth one of the members of the council would say something along the lines of, 'It's all right for you white mob, you've been killing us black mob for 210 years. Why should we listen to you now?" The most prominent of these dissidents was an imposing Aboriginal man from the Kimberley, Arnold "Puggy" Hunter. He was chair of the National Aboriginal Community Controlled Health Organisations (NACCHO). This was the umbrella organisation for most of the Aboriginal health centres which were controlled by Aboriginal boards formed from the local community. NACCHO was not uniformly accepted as the voice for such organisations, particularly those located in North Queensland and the Cape York area, where Torres Strait Islanders were more numerous. Not much progress was made in that first session. I was formally introduced to Puggy at morning tea by Ian Anderson, the University of Melbourne's first Indigenous medical graduate. Disarmingly, he said, 'Don't worry about that stuff this morning, Richard. I've got my electorate I have to play to too, you know'. And he was right. Later he invited me to a meeting of the NACCHO executive, and politics there was really tough and direct.

As the meetings progressed, I developed considerable sympathy for many of the views put forward forcibly by the Indigenous members of council. They spoke of all the waste which occurred when well-meaning bureaucrats responded to an identified health problem by addressing that problem directly and without adequate consultation with the Indigenous communities affected. Examples cited included cervical cancer screening programs and screening for eye complications of diabetes with retinal cameras. It was stated that the department of health introduced screening and treatment programs in remote communities and because they had not been adequately integrated into the primary care system, they were poorly attended and later withdrawn as failures.

'Helicopter' researchers were also a source of considerable angst. The term referred to researchers from universities and hospitals located far away from the communities who did research on the communities' problems, published the research often without discussing it with the local community and then flew off with their career prospects enhanced but without benefit for the communities.

Other concerns that the Indigenous members held about research were the source of frustration for me. They questioned the value of data collection and analysis. They felt they knew what the problems were and it was time to get on and solve them. A reasonable point, but at the end of the day, careful baseline and progressive data collection is vital to the development and implementation of the most effective programs to address the problems.

CHAPTER 16

There was a deep suspicion of any genetic research. At the time, there was a large world effort to attempt to understand more of the origin and migration patterns of homo sapiens. The concerns about this study were that the information may be used to decide how 'Aboriginal' someone might be and therefore determine their entitlement to some special benefits available to Indigenous people and, secondly, that it might be designed to show the relative degree of primitiveness of different racial groups. Concern about this study was soon generalised to all forms of genetic research and to a deep suspicion of NHMRC itself. I spent quite a lot of time trying to explain potential benefits of such research, detailing ethical safeguards and indicating the strong commitment NHMRC had to improving Indigenous health through relevant research done in partnership with Indigenous communities. Specific ethical guidelines now apply to such research.

There was a sad postscript to the Puggy Hunter story. At a later meeting of the National Aboriginal and Torres Strait Islander Health Council, Puggy was making a point strongly and, to enhance the dramatic impact, he added, 'Anyway, you won't have to worry about me for much longer. I'm fifty-three and that's past the use-by date for a blackfella'. He was right. A few months later, he was found dead by the side of a road in the Kimberley, having suffered a heart attack. Like many other Indigenous people of his age, he had the combination of diabetes, renal failure and coronary artery disease. These non-communicable diseases are major contributors to the shortened lifespan of Indigenous people, which remains at about fifteen years less than that of non-Indigenous Australians. Increased susceptibility to these non-communicable diseases is shared by many other traditional communities which have made the transition from a 'hunter-gatherer' lifestyle to a more sedentary lifestyle, with readily available processed food and drink rich in saturated fat, sugar and salt.

I was privileged to meet a number of outstanding Indigenous leaders in my role with NHMRC and NATSIHC. I do not pretend to understand all the issues and complexities affecting Indigenous health, but a number of conclusions are very clear. First, substantial improvement will depend on developing strong partnerships with Indigenous communities. It may be a slow process, but it is essential for progress. Second, health cannot be isolated from other areas of Indigenous disadvantage, such as education, housing, meaningful employment, healthy diets, physical activity and cultural pride. Third, given the extent to which mainstream services are under-utilised by Indigenous people, there is the need either for substantial additional investment in specific programs directed to Indigenous people and developed with them or, alternatively, considerable change to mainstream services so that they are more culturally appropriate for Indigenous people as well as other people from culturally different backgrounds.

There are many people, both Indigenous and non-Indigenous, doing outstanding work in these areas, and although it is frustratingly slow, there is evidence of improvement in a number of parameters. Notably, neonatal mortality rates have decreased markedly, the incidence and outcomes of infectious diseases have improved and the potential epidemic of HIV-AIDS has not eventuated. Although there is still a big discrepancy compared with the non-Indigenous population, life expectancy has increased significantly. More Indigenous people than ever before are able to access appropriate services for chronic disease such as renal failure. Although there are many exceptions, many Aboriginal communities are successfully combating problems related to alcohol and other drugs and domestic violence.

Chapter 17

PRESIDENT OF THE ROYAL AUSTRALASIAN COLLEGE OF PHYSICIANS

After finishing my term as chair of the NHMRC, I was elected to the position of president of the Royal Australasian College of Physicians (RACP). Initially, this college comprised doctors trained in all the sub-specialty areas of internal medicine, ranging from general medicine through cardiology, rheumatology, endocrinology, neurology, gastroenterology, thoracic medicine and so on. In recent years, related but separate medical specialties had agreed to join the college as faculties. These are public health medicine, occupational and environmental medicine and rehabilitation medicine. Although responsibility for overseeing the training program and examinations for admission to gaining specialist status had resided with the college, there had been a separate College of Paediatrics which had agreed to cease its independent existence and become a division of the college. Later, specialty chapters were formed within the college structure with chapters of palliative medicine, addiction medicine, sexual health medicine and community child health. The RACP had become a large and diverse organisation responsible for the training, examination and continuing professional development of over 13,000 specialist medical practitioners.

I had had an active involvement in the affairs of the college for many years. I was appointed to the board of censors (soon to become the committee for examinations) in 1978 and had remained as an examiner until I completed a term as the chair of the committee for examinations and chairman of the board of censors in 1990. I held many other positions, including chair of the Asia Pacific committee, a member of the Aboriginal and Torres Strait Islander committee and chairman of the Victorian state committee, as well as vice-president and deputy president.

NEW TRICKS

The RACP had been established by a group of physicians (specialists in internal medicine) in 1938 to improve the quality of medical practice and to increase knowledge through research. These objectives have matured and expanded. Amongst other objectives, the current constitution of the college defines the following aims: 'to promote the highest quality medical care and patient safety through education training and assessment, to educate and train the next generation of physicians, to maintain professional standards and ethics, to increase the evidence and knowledge on which the practice of physicians is based through research and dissemination of new knowledge and innovation to the profession and community' and 'to seek improved health for all people by developing and advocating health and social policy in partnership with health consumers and jurisdictions'.

Clearly this is a broad remit. The expansion of the college to include the paediatricians, the faculties and the chapters greatly expanded the range of expertise available within the college. Until the 1990s, the role of the college had very much been around the examination of potential physicians and paediatricians and the accreditation of training programs for the subspecialist phase of training (the advanced training programs). There had been initiatives, driven by individuals such as Sir 'Jock' Frew, Bryan Hudson and Sir Kenneth Noad to build links with Asia, particularly Singapore, and there are many college fellows in Asia who view with gratitude the training they received in Australia. There had also been active efforts to provide physician training to medical practitioners from Papua New Guinea and the college administered an AusAID program designed to provide training for medical officers (and later nurses) in Australia. Sporadic efforts had been made to engage with the health issues in Australian and New Zealand indigenous communities. Although individual college fellows were making major contributions in this area, the college as a whole found it difficult to play an effective role. Some funding was available to provide small travel grants to Australian and New Zealand physicians and advanced trainees to undertake research overseas, but the support for research was minimal. The college conducted an annual meeting and, through its state and New Zealand committees, interacted with the state health jurisdictions to improve training opportunities and to advocate in relation to health policy and health care delivery in the states. Overall, however, the focus of the college was very much on the examination of physicians and the accreditation of training programs.

CHAPTER 17

Things changed markedly under the presidency of John Chalmers, a dynamic and highly intelligent physician who had been the foundation professor of medicine at the Flinders University medical school. He had recruited around him an outstanding group of young physician researchers, which enabled Flinders Medical Centre very quickly to become one of the leading teaching hospitals in the country, with integration of the university and hospital staff in a creative partnership designed to deliver the highest quality clinical care, teaching and research.

Chalmers felt that although the college had done an excellent job in examination and specialist training programs and accreditation, its efforts in research had been inadequate. He felt there was a real need for the college to show leadership to ensure that a significant proportion of our young physicians would go on to undertake research training and become physician researchers. This would require the college to have significant funds, which it could apply judiciously to encourage physician trainees to undertake research training and also to allow those physicians who had completed a research degree and had perhaps had some research training overseas to become established as independent researchers and demonstrate their ability to attract ongoing research funding from bodies such as the NHMRC.

Under Chalmers' leadership, the college council established the Research and Education Foundation and undertook a major fundraising campaign to provide it with meaningful funds to allow the college to have an impact. Chalmers believed that the college could only expect substantial contributions from the corporate sector if the fellows themselves demonstrated their commitment by making personal donations. Fellows were recruited to ask their colleagues to contribute, a new approach for the college, and Chalmers and others approached potential corporate donors, particularly from the pharmaceutical industry.

This initiative has been very successful. John persuaded Ken Roberts, the then chairman and managing director of Wellcome Australasia to chair the Research and Education Foundation Board, and he held that position until I succeeded him in 2009. The foundation had grown to a corpus of well over AUS$30 million and now awards over fifty research grants per year, focusing on research entry awards and early career researchers, particularly working at the interface between basic science and its clinical translation (or the public health equivalent).

Another area where the college had been less effective than it might have been was in 'developing and advocating health and social policy in partnership with health consumers and jurisdictions'. Recognising the importance of this area to the health of people in Australia and New Zealand, the college council decided to form the Health Policy Unit in 1995. I was involved in the appointment of its foundation director, Craig Patterson. Craig was a young lawyer who had worked in the commonwealth department of health and had served on committees devising policies relating to HIV-AIDS. He was a flamboyant character, highly intelligent and openly gay. It was an inspired choice for the college.

The deserved reputation of the college was that it was conservative, and although it was respected for its role in educating and maintaining standards of physicians, its ability to connect with the general community was considered to be inadequate. While it was listened to politely by politicians, its ability to influence policy was limited. Craig had an inimitable ability to connect with consumer organisations and with health bureaucrats and made the college a much more effective organisation in influencing government policy. The unit has now been restyled the College Policy and Advocacy Committee and has expert advisory groups on therapeutics, workforce, rural health, Aboriginal and Torres Strait Islander and Maori Health and eHealth. It has been responsible for a number of policies, position statements and submissions. It has as its guiding principle that wherever possible, all its publications and statements are evidence-based.

During my time as president, one of its major policy statements related to illicit drugs. The policy was very much based around a harm-minimisation approach rather than law enforcement. It argued that the current 'zero tolerance' policy favoured by the conservative government in Australia as well as by the United States of America had clearly failed with many deaths from drug overdose, rising rates of hepatitis C and to a lesser extent HIV-AIDS from shared injecting needles and much crime being associated with drugs, either their illegal importation, manufacture or trafficking, or in breaking and entering, personal assaults or other illegal attempts to obtain money to support drug habits. The college policy argued for better education, treatment and rehabilitation facilities, with more training positions for specialists in the field. Other recommendations included trials of supervised heroin-injecting facilities, medically prescribed and supervised heroin treatment for defined addicts and easier access to opioid

CHAPTER 17

substitution therapy. Education and treatment, rather than imprisonment, were supported for users of drugs.

The policy was launched by Reverend Tim Costello, one of the leading social commentators on social justice issues and later CEO of World Vision. Its recommendations were largely in line with the recommendations of the Premier's Drug Advisory Council in Victoria established by Jeff Kennett and chaired by David Penington. Both this council's recommendations and those of the college, although viewed by some as being radical, were in line with practice that had been proved to be effective in countries such as Switzerland and later implemented in a number of other countries.

The prime minister, John Howard, had deeply conservative views of the issues and these were reinforced by an advisory committee the prime minister had established, chaired by Major Brian Watters of the New South Wales Salvation Army. Under this advice, the commonwealth was adopting a strong law enforcement approach using terms such as 'war on drugs' from the Nixon and Reagan eras. However, although the expenditure on law enforcement still vastly and inappropriately exceeded the expenditure on education, treatment and other harm-minimisation approaches, there has been a considerably increased recognition of the need for and relative effectiveness of harm-minimisation approaches. Diversion from the justice system to education and treatment for drug users is now commonplace in both state and the federal jurisdictions.

The advocacy of the college as well as the public leadership of David Penington, Alex Wodak and others have certainly helped to shift the balance to a greater extent towards harm minimisation, although there is still much need for improved treatment and rehabilitation programs and better approaches to other aspects of harm minimisation, such as opioid substitution, medically supervised heroin prescription and supply, supervised injecting facilities and needle-exchange programs in prisons. Although by no means an expert, I was much informed by my role in promoting the college position. More recently, I have had the privilege of chairing an expert advisory group advising the Victorian government on its strategy for reducing the adverse impact of alcohol and other drugs. Despite the populist 'zero tolerance' rhetoric, much progress is being made in the harm-minimisation area.

The college also played an active role in advocacy about health issues relating to asylum seekers who had arrived by sea and were being held in detention centres often for long periods. The mental health effects on children, in particular, were the topic of a presentation at a college meeting. Advocacy by people such as Professor Louise Newman, a child psychiatrist who spoke at the meeting, has led to a change in policy concerning children in detention, although a great deal of further reform is needed.

The college's greater effectiveness in the area of advocacy was very largely due to the inspirational leadership of Craig Patterson. Craig was later CEO of the College of Psychiatrists and returned to be CEO of the Royal Australasian College of Physicians. He died suddenly and tragically at a young age. He had shown the college that it could be an effective voice in health issues of concern to the community and that it needed to engage with others, including consumer groups to be effective in doing so.

International engagement, particularly with South-East Asia, had over the last three decades or so been a major interest of the leaders of the college. Many of the leading physicians in Singapore and, to a lesser extent, Malaysia and Hong Kong, had had a period of postgraduate training in Australia, often as a prelude to sitting the membership examination and later becoming fellows at the college. Changes to the training requirements in the 1970s, with three years of supervised advanced training being required before admission to fellowship, had made it much more difficult for doctors from outside Australia and New Zealand to satisfy the requirements for fellowship of the college, thus lessening the links with the academies of medicine in Singapore, Malaysia and the more recently formed academy in Hong Kong. Meanwhile, the less-constrained conditions pertaining to membership of the UK colleges of physicians led to many young doctors seeking that pathway.

Considerable efforts were made during my presidency to rebuild the links and to build strong links also with the Royal College of Physicians of Thailand. Joint scientific meetings were held and relationships were warm, but it is inevitable, with the greater sophistication of medical training and practice, that the qualifications administered by the host country would increasingly be seen as the most relevant for specialist practice in that country. Our emphasis instead was on encouraging exchange of young doctors between our countries to build international links and partnerships rather than expecting many to become fellows of our college.

Being president of the RACP leads to the receipt of a number of honorary fellowships of international medical colleges or academies. On one such occasion, I was guest lecturer at the Ceylon College of Physicians and was

CHAPTER 17

awarded honorary fellowship in a moving ceremony. Sri Lanka has managed to preserve high quality medical education and practice despite the devastating social and economic impact of their prolonged civil war.

The most spectacular event of this nature was the award of Honorary Fellowship of the Royal College of Physicians of Thailand. The award was presented by HRH Princess Chulabhorn, who has an impressive academic record as a chemist and is an advocate for scientific research. The royal family is revered in Thailand, and we were required to kneel on the stage, ensuring our head stayed lower than the princess's. It was harder for me than for my Thai counterpart, Supachai Chaithiraphan, who was about 155 cm tall. He became a good friend.

At a celebratory dinner afterwards, it became clear that Caroline and I were expected to sing for our hosts. Karaoke was taken very seriously by the Thais, and we were told that most of the Thais were receiving singing lessons. Supachai and his colleagues were very impressive. When our turn came, we asked the band to play 'Waltzing Matilda'. We were met with looks of bemusement. We struggled on. I had a vague idea of the words beyond the first verse but no idea of the tune. Caroline had a vague idea of the tune but no idea of the words. We sat down to muted applause and considerable embarrassment. Still, I think they appreciated us having a go.

At one of the RACP annual ceremonies when I was president, the council, at my suggestion, invited Mechai Viravaidya to be the Sir Arthur Mills Orator at the ceremony. Mechai is a larger-than-life figure who gained fame when, as a member of the Thai parliament, he campaigned strongly for birth control using condoms. Under his inspiring leadership, the average Thai family size fell from 7 to 1.5 children. With the HIV-AIDS epidemic, Mechai (by now commonly known as Mr Condom) urged the use of condoms once more to prevent the spread of the virus. He gave a very lively lecture and finished by distributing condoms in a variety of novelty arrangements to the audience. I am sure that would have been a first for the college ceremony.

Attending meetings of sister colleges, getting to know the medical leaders and learning of the problems and solutions relating to medical education and practice in countries around the world was an enjoyable and enlightening experience.

A universal problem was that of excessive subspecialisation. The general physician (internist) was becoming an endangered species. Instead, physicians were training and practising as cardiologists, neurologists, gastroenterologists, endocrinologists, rheumatologists, infectious diseases specialists, thoracic physicians, haematologists or oncologists. In addition to the decreasing numbers training as general physicians, only paediatricians and geriatricians looked after whole individuals in normal circumstances. Rehabilitation specialists, occupational health physicians, intensivists and palliative care physicians dealt with the whole person, but only in special circumstances. Special societies had grown up around the organ and system subspecialists. The college was seen as the large faceless body responsible for guarding the entrance to specialist practice with their examination system and then imposing training requirements and fees that were often seen as restrictive and expensive.

Once physicians had completed their advanced training, they felt a much stronger relationship with their special society, attended the special society meetings and read the specialist journals. The college seemed distant and irrelevant and yet continued to demand annual subscriptions generally far higher than those of the special society. Not surprisingly, talk of secession recurred amongst the special societies, particularly the larger and more wealthy , such as the Cardiac Society.

I was invited to debate the role of the college versus that of the special society at a meeting of the Cardiac Society. I argued that being part of a larger body with accepted standards of examination and training, an accepted continuing education program and a high profile because of advocacy around inequities in health and other areas of social justice, was a great protection for the cardiologists.

If they were to stand alone and set up their own entry and training standards, accusations of restrictive trade practice would be hard to defend. Moreover, the high earnings attracted by interventional cardiologists would be starkly revealed and again hard to defend without accusations of self-interest. I won the day on that occasion, but the issue of making the college relevant to its very broad constituency is and will continue to be an ongoing challenge for future generations of office bearers. Meanwhile, I am convinced that there continues to be a real need for general physicians. General practitioners frequently seek a broad overview of patients with multiple problems or general systemic symptoms which cannot be confidently ascribed to a particular system. Similarly, surgeons and anaesthetists often require the reassurance of a general physician before operating on the frail

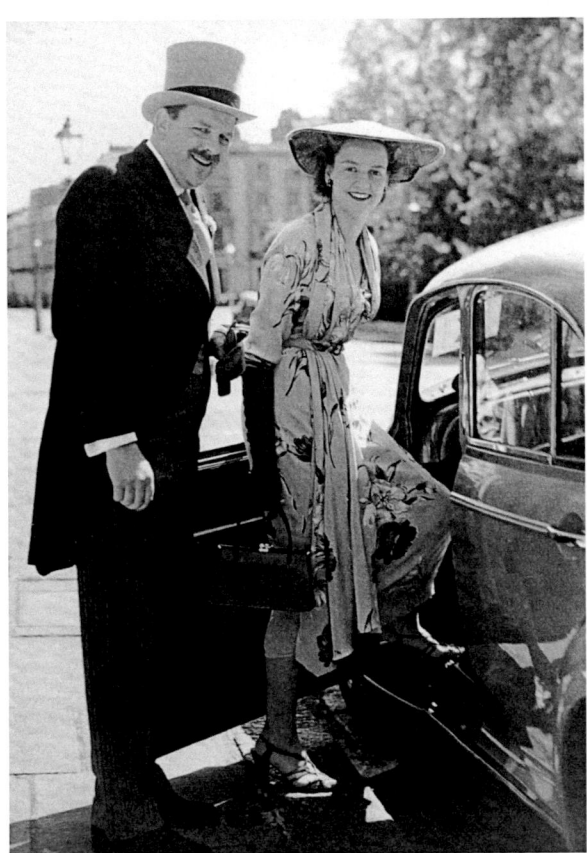

Left: **My parents, Graeme and Peg Larkins, off to Buckingham Palace for Queen Elizabeth's garden party, 1953.**

Below: **Admission to the bar for my mother, Peg Lusink, 1966.**

Left to right: Theo Lusink (my stepfather), Joan Rosanove QC (my grandmother), Peg Lusink, John Larkins (my older brother).

Both photos from the author's personal collection.

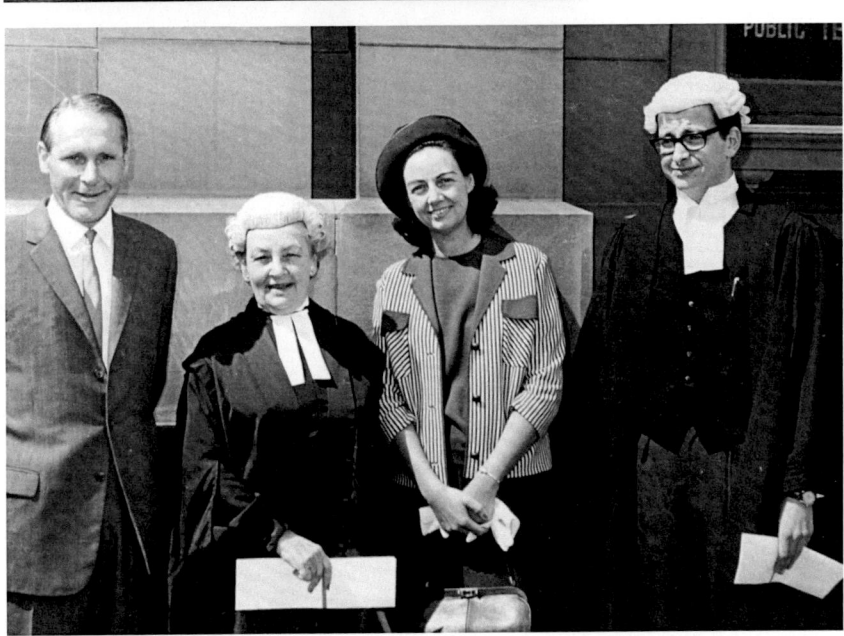

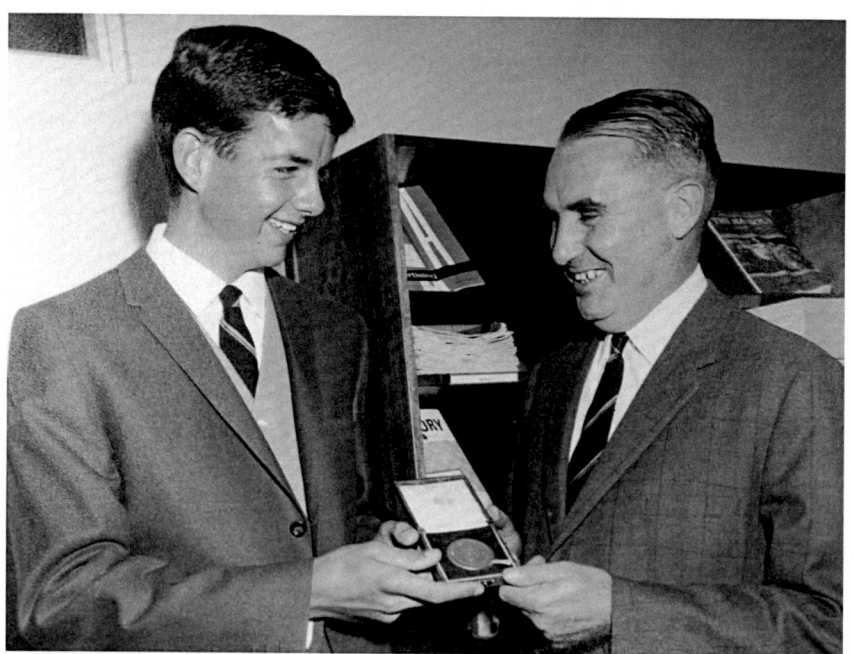

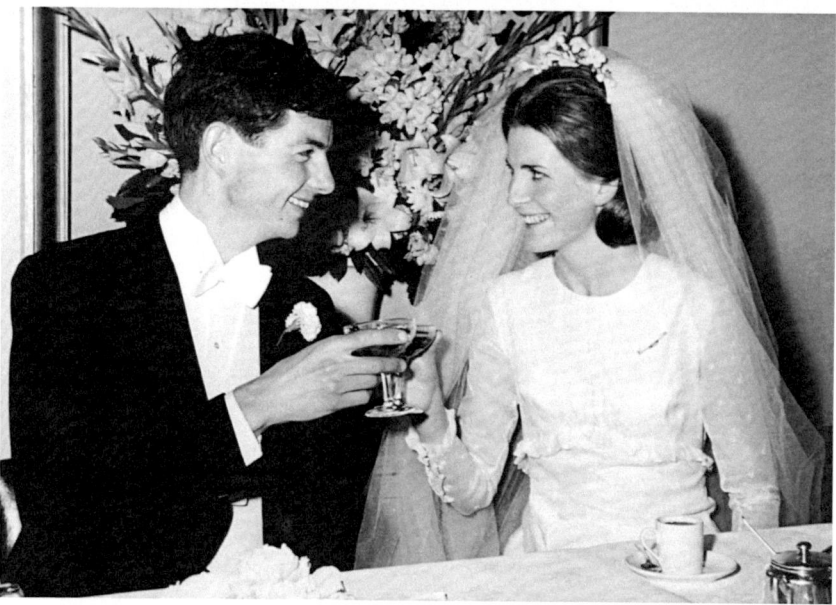

Top: **Presentation of BHP medal for top of Victoria at matriculation in physics, chemistry and a branch of maths by Sir Ian McLennan, Chairman of BHP, 1960.**

Above: **Wedding dinner, 7 December 1966.**

Both photos from the author's personal collection.

OBESE MICE ASSIST IN RESEARCH

Research which could one day shed light on the development of diabetes is being conducted by two doctors of the University of Melbourne Department of Medicine and the Royal Melbourne Hospital.

Doctor R. G. Larkins and Doctor F. I. R. Martin have just had a paper published in the British scientific journal, "Nature".

In the paper, they describe research work they have done with a strain of mice that develops obesity and diabetes.

The mice, originally bred in New Zealand, become abnormally fat and develop an obese defect of their pancreas, the organ which normally makes insulin.

Doctor Larkins and Doctor Martin have found that the mice cannot respond to raised levels of sugar or other agents in the blood, which normally cause insulin to be secreted.

However, they do respond dramatically to the simple substance, arginine — an amino acid normally present in the body.

The doctors say their findings so far have no direct application to the treatment of human diabetes. But they do lead to important implications concerning the normal mechanism by which insulin may be released from the pancreas.

The observation also raises the previously unsuspected possibility that, with increasing weight gain and obesity, the nature of the pancreas' response to different stimuli may change.

The work of the two doctors in Melbourne has been supported by the National Health and Medical Research Council of Australia.

As well, Dr. Larkins was the recipient of the Sheppard M. Lowe Scholarship from the University of Melbourne and a grant from the Victor Hurley Research Fund, Royal Melbourne Hospital.

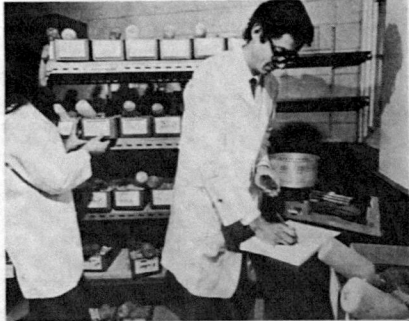

Dr. Larkins and Laboratory Technician, Lilly Simenova, at work in the laboratory. Dr. Larkins is holding one of the overweight mice in his hand.

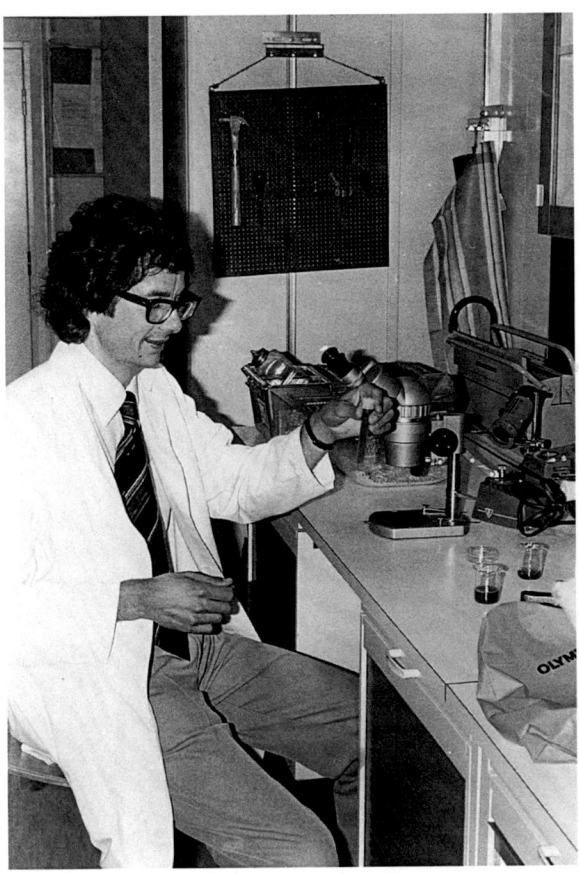

Above: **First venture in research, 1971.**

Published in *Royal Melbourne Life News*, clipping held in author's personal collection.

Left: **Isolating pancreatic islets in Uppsala, Sweden, 1974.**

Personal collection.

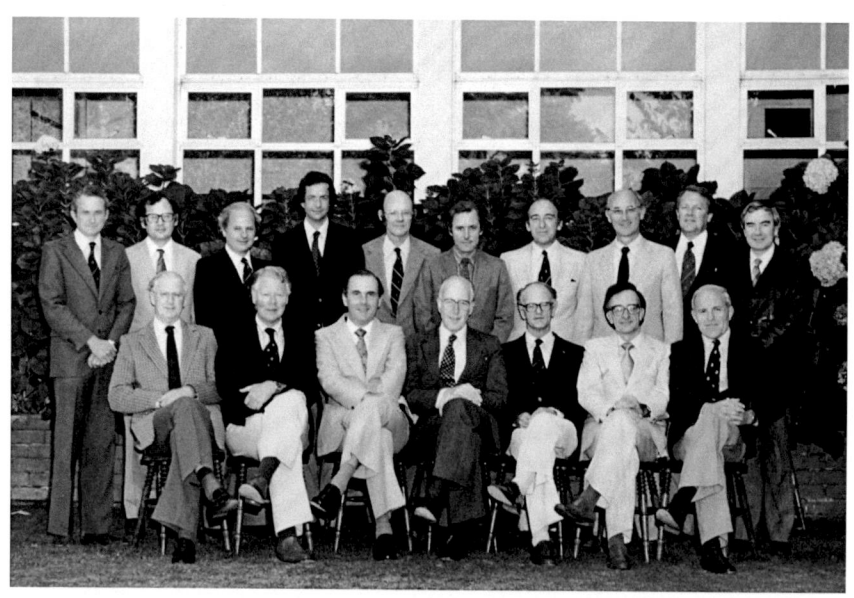

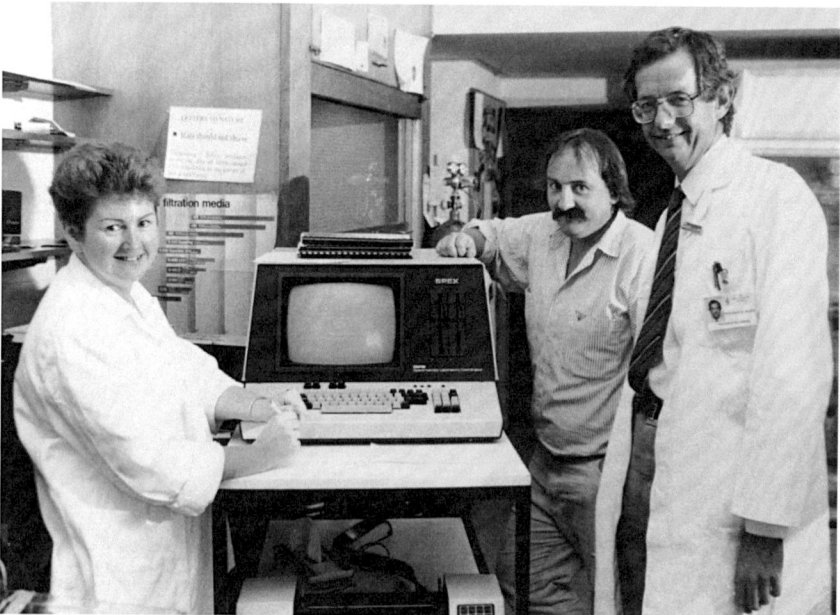

Top: **Committee for Examinations, Royal Australasian College of Physicians, 1979.**
Back row (l–r): Dick Kimber, Don Chisholm, John Chalmers, Richard Larkins, David Tiller, Graeme Morgan, Alex Cohen, Peter Castaldi, Bernard Gilligan, Ray Tiernan. Front row (l–r): Tom Robertson, John Turtle, Maurice Clark, John Beveridge, Laurie Powell, Ken Perkins.

Above: **Marjorie Dunlop and Michael Hill at the Department of Medicine, Royal Melbourne Hospital, 1987.**
Both photos from author's personal collection.

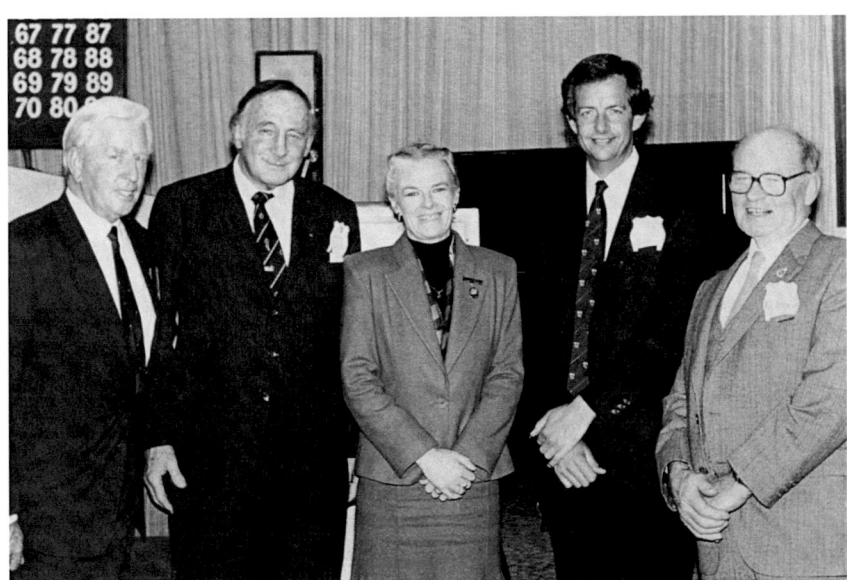

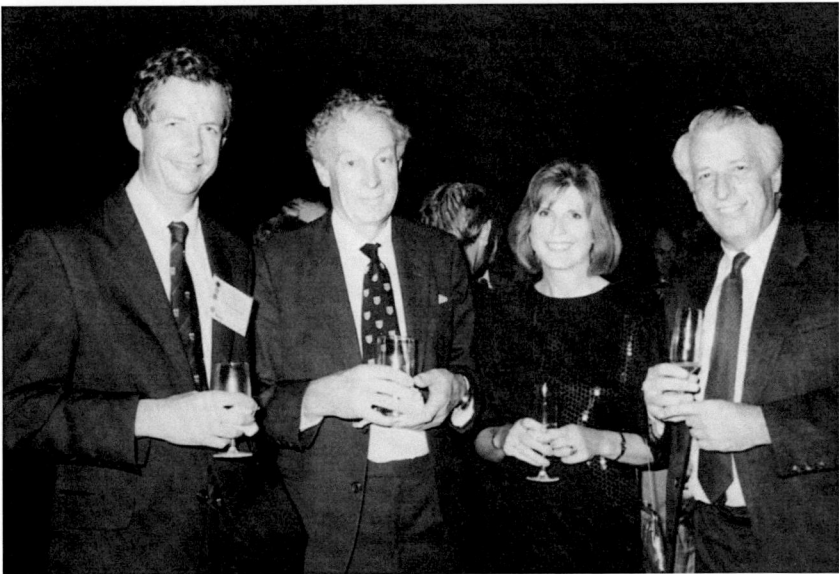

Top: **Spruiking the Sir Edward Dunlop Medical Research Fund at Essendon RSL, 17 July 1988.**

Left to right: Ray Wheeler, Sir Edward Dunlop, Councillor Monica Hayes, Joe Beaumont.

Above: **At a dinner celebrating the golden jubilee of the Royal Australasian College of Physicians, 1988.**

Left to right: Richard Larkins, Ken Fairley, Caroline Larkins, Gus Nossal.

Both photos from author's private collection.

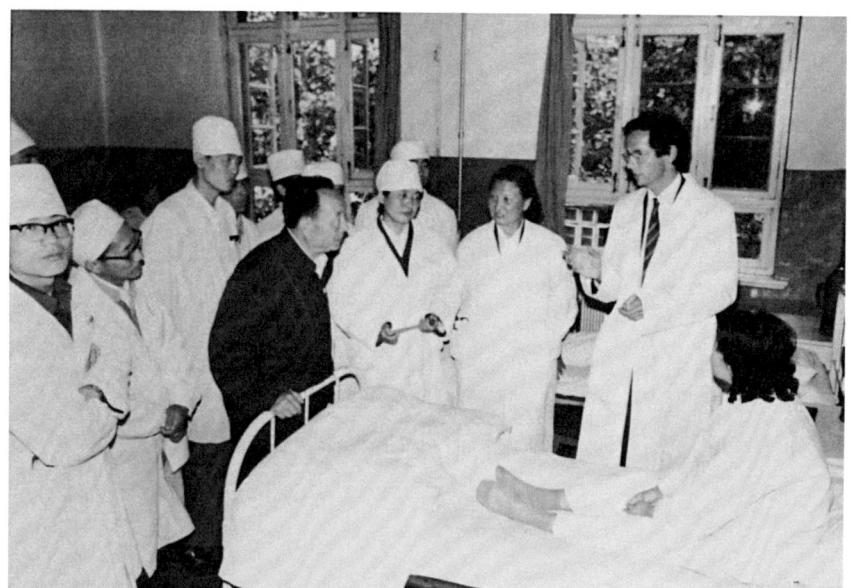

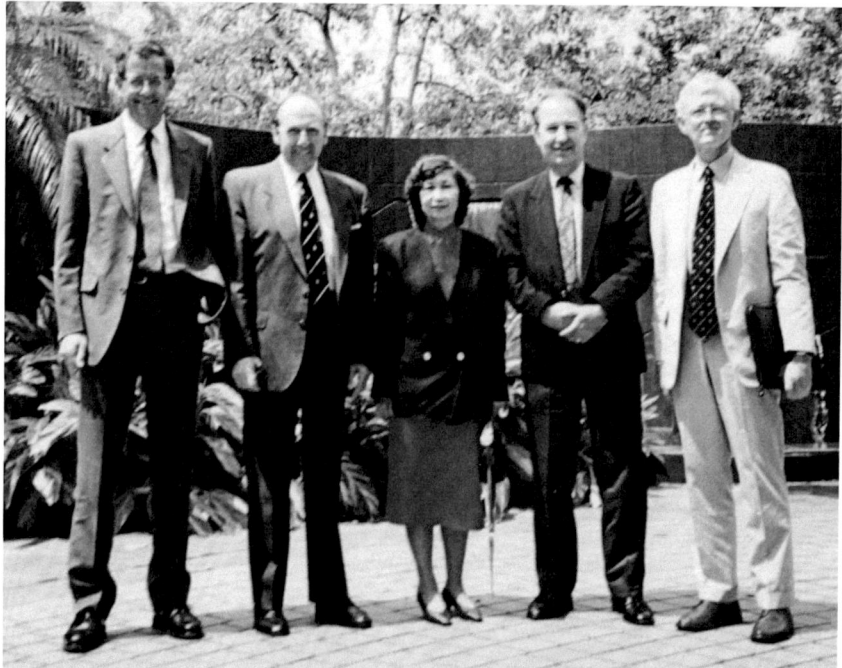

Top: **Shandong Affiliated Hospital, 1985.**
Bedside teaching, China style.

Above: **In Hong Kong, on delegation from Royal Australasian College of Physicians.**
Left to right: Richard Larkins, Alex Cohen, Rosie Young, Peter Procopis, Don Cameron.
Both photos from author's personal collection.

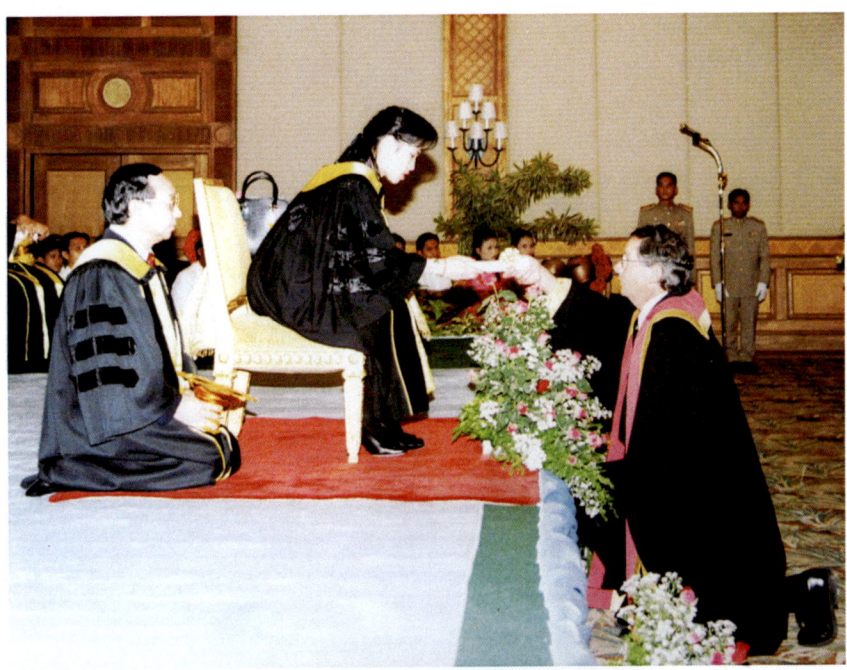

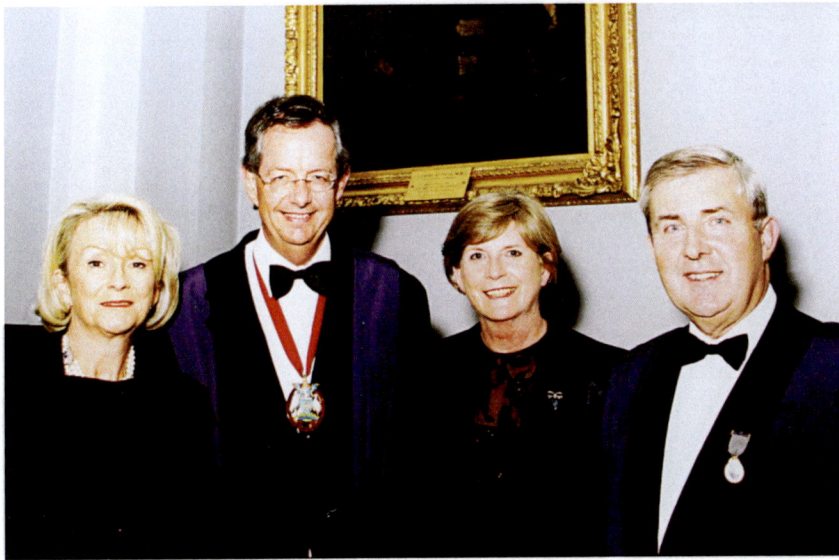

Top: **Bestowal of honorary fellowship of the Royal College of Physicians of Thailand, 2002, by Princess Chulabhorn.**

Above: **At the time of the conferral of Fellowship of Physicians of Ireland (RCPI).**

Left to right: Mary Keogh, Richard Larkins, Caroline Larkins, Brian Keogh (immediate past president of the RCPI).

Both photos from author's personal collection.

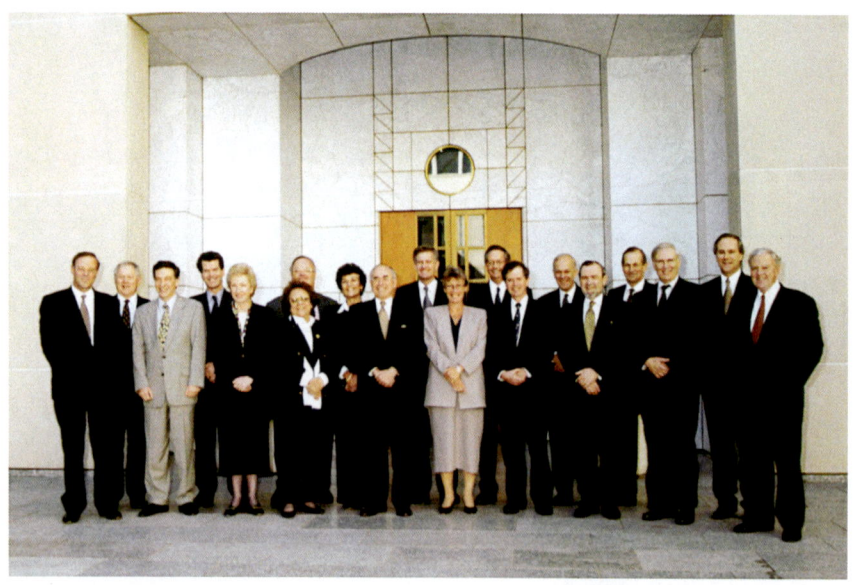

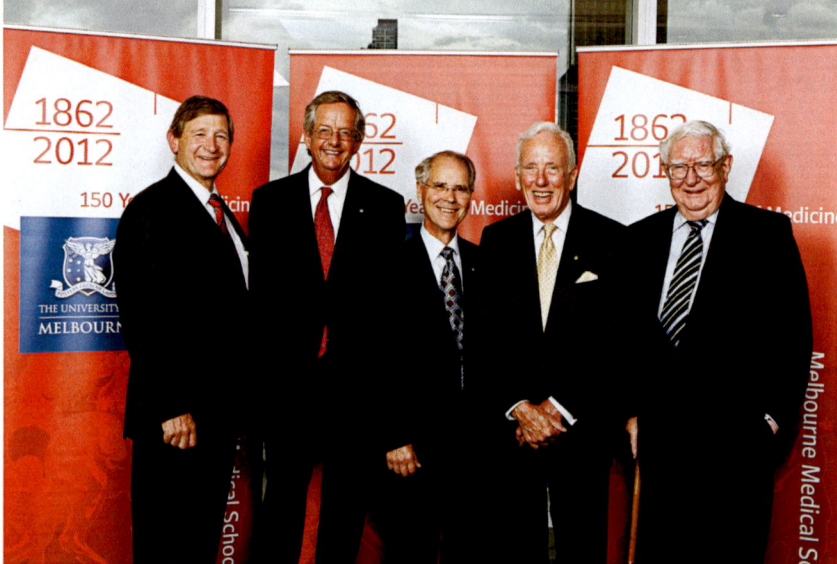

Top: **Inaugural meeting of Prime Minister's Science, Engineering and Innovation Council (PMSEIC), 29 May 1998.**

Photo by AUSPIC.

Above: **The inaugural recipients of the Brownless Medal – all the living deans of the medical school, 15 March 2012.**

Left to right: James Angus, Richard Larkins, Graeme Ryan, David Penington, George Clunie.

Courtesy of *Chiron*, 2012, Melbourne Medical School 150th Anniversary edition.

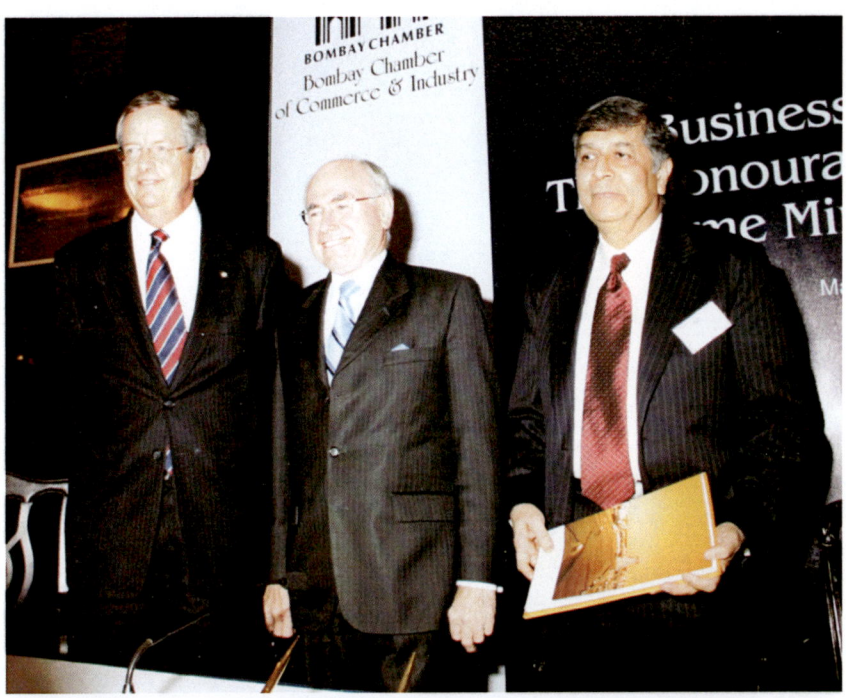

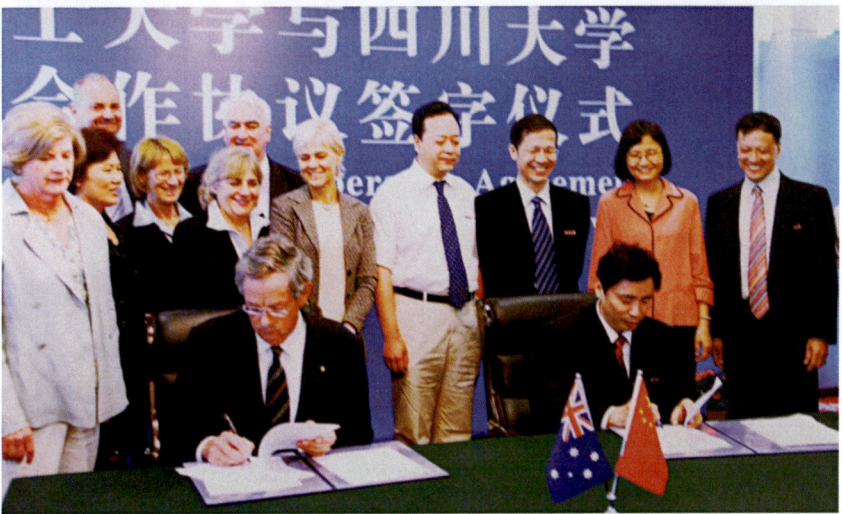

Top: **The signing of the MOU in Mumbai to establish the Indian Institute of Technology and Monash University Research Academy, 2006.**

Left to right: Richard Larkins, Prime Minister John Howard, Ashok Misra, the director of the Indian Institute of Technology, Bombay.

Personal collection.

Above: **Signing the MOU with Sichuan University, with President Hie Xie Ping.**

Courtesy of Sichuan University.

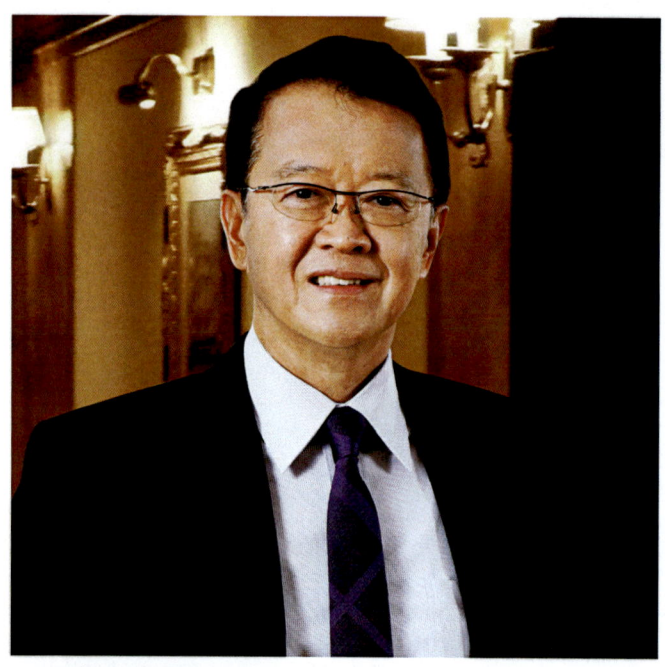

Left: **Dr Tan Sri Jeffrey Cheah AO.**

Photo courtesy of Sunway Group.

Below: **Monash Sunway campus, Malaysia, 2008.**

Photographer: Mark Rogers. Monash University Archives, IN7443.

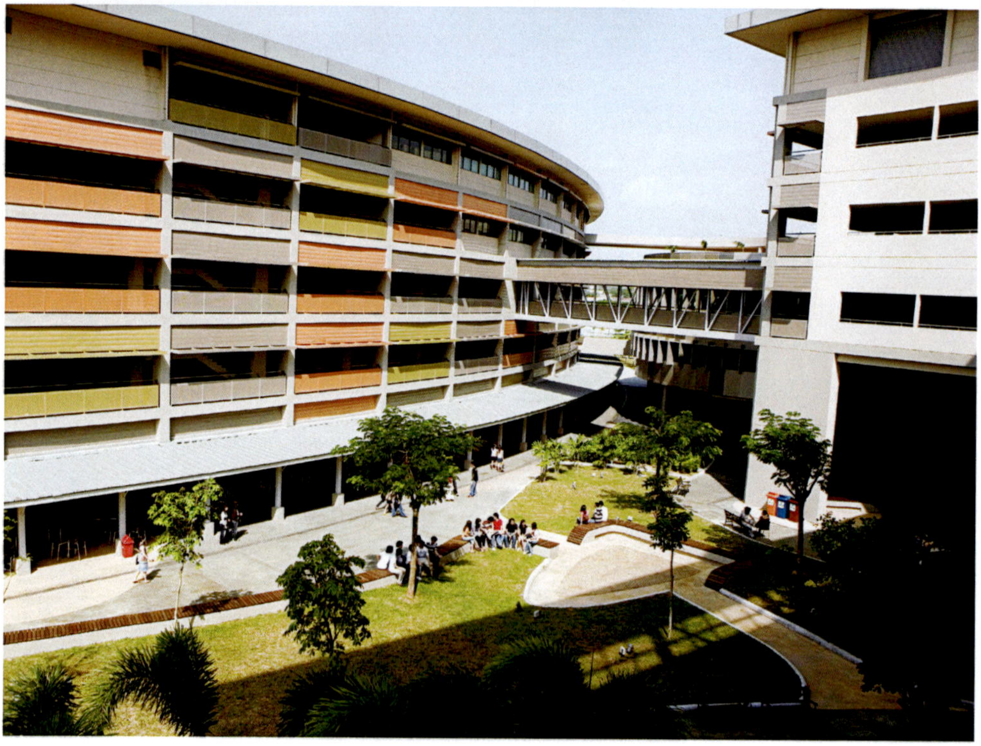

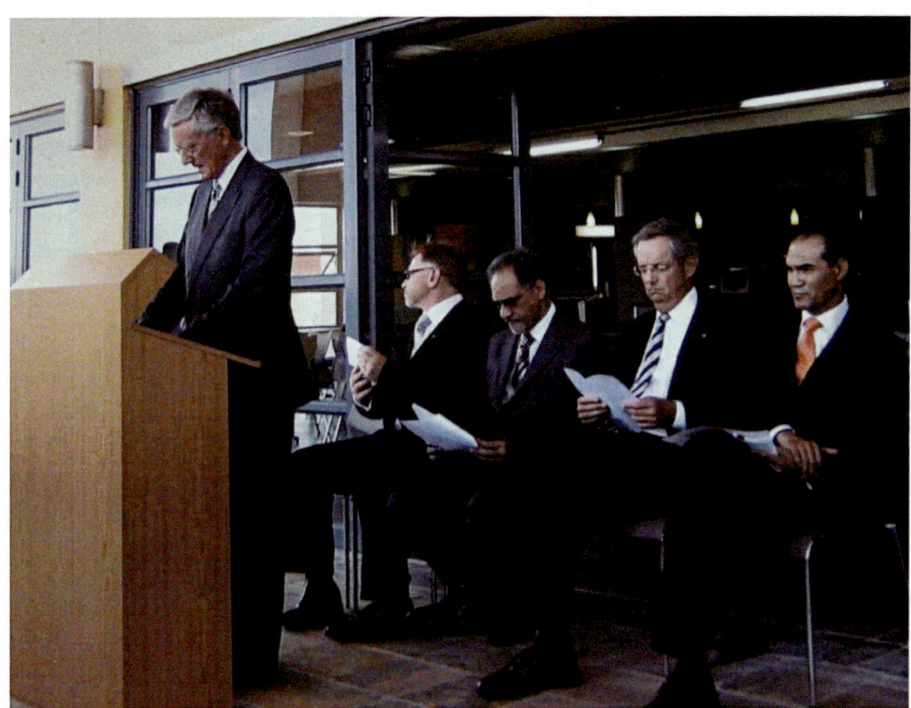

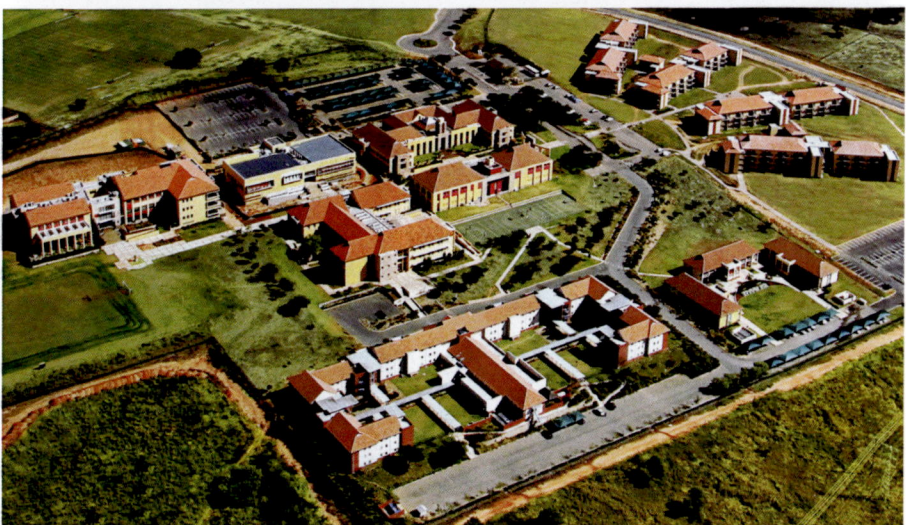

Top: **Opening of the library and learning commons, Monash South Africa.**
Left to right: Chancellor Jerry Ellis at the podium; His Excellency Philip Green, Australia's high commissioner to South Africa; the deputy minister for education; Richard Larkins; Tyrone Pretorius.

Above: **Aerial view of Monash South Africa, 2009.**
This photo was presented to me as a farewell gift from Monash South Africa.
Both photos from author's personal collection.

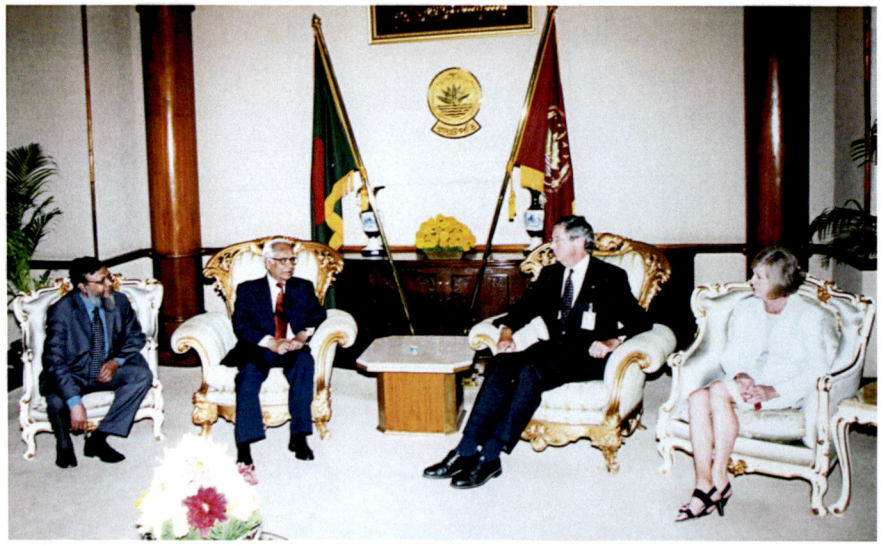

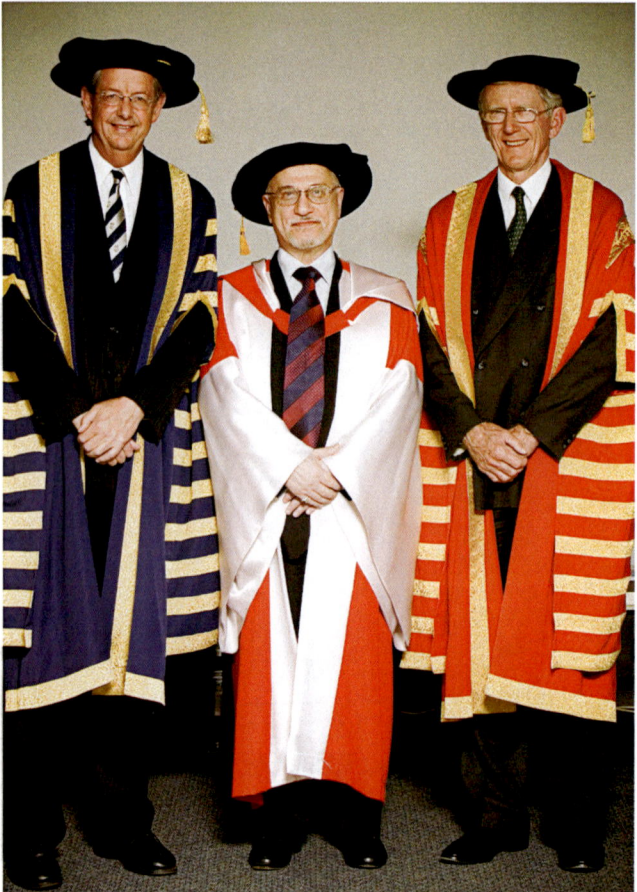

Above: **With the president of Bangladesh, Professor Iajuddin Ahmed, at the Presidental Palace in February 2006.**

Personal collection.

Left: **Richard Larkins (left), with Hussain Al-Shahristani and Chancellor Mr Jerry Ellis after the award of honorary Doctor of Laws to Hussain Al-Shahristani, 2006.**

Photographer: Greg Ford. Monash University Archives, IN8003.

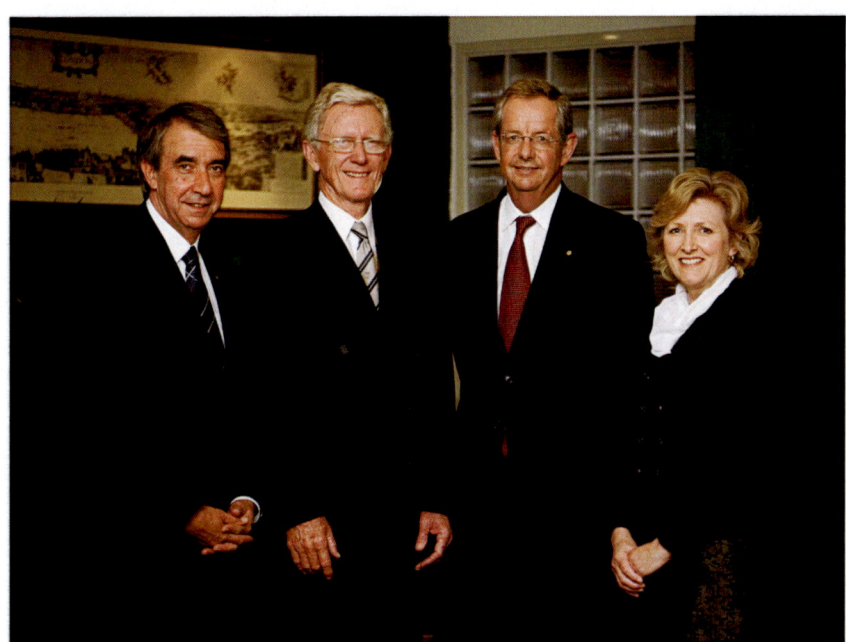

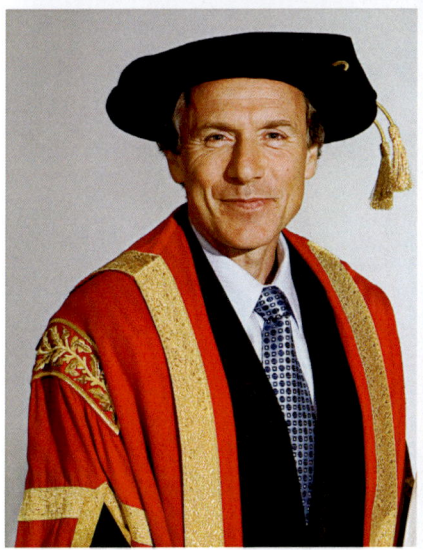
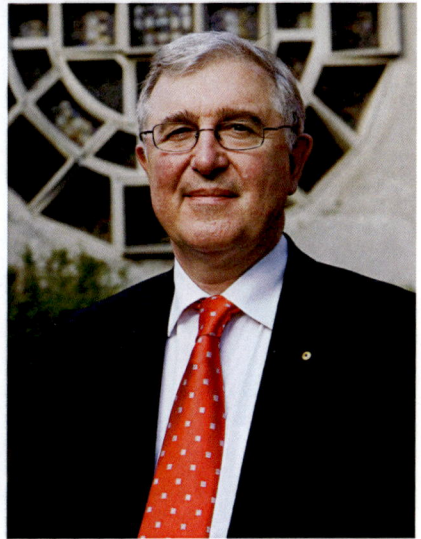

Top: **Chancellor Jerry Ellis's farewell in 2007.**

Left to right: Deputy Chancellor Paul Ramler, Chancellor Jerry Ellis, Vice-Chancellor Professor Richard Larkins and Deputy Chancellor Dr Leanne Rowe at the chancellor's farewell.

Above left: **Chancellor Dr Alan Finkel, 2008.**

Above right: **Vice-Chancellor Professor Edward Byrne, 2009.**

Photographer: Greg Ford. Monash University Archives, IN8384, IN8008 and IN8326.

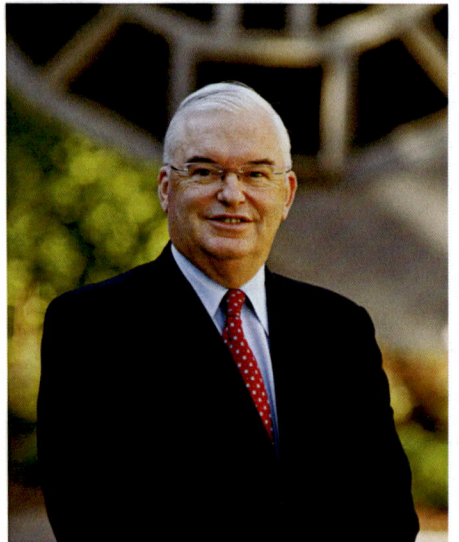
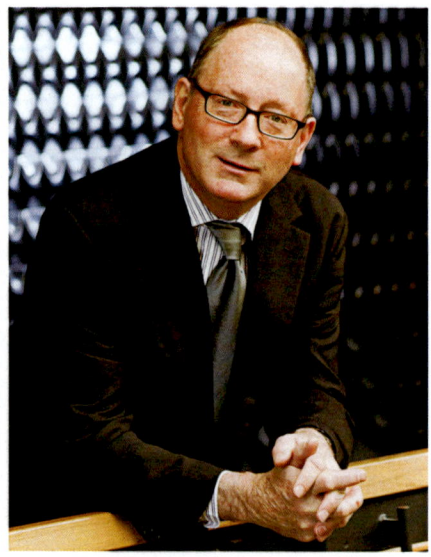
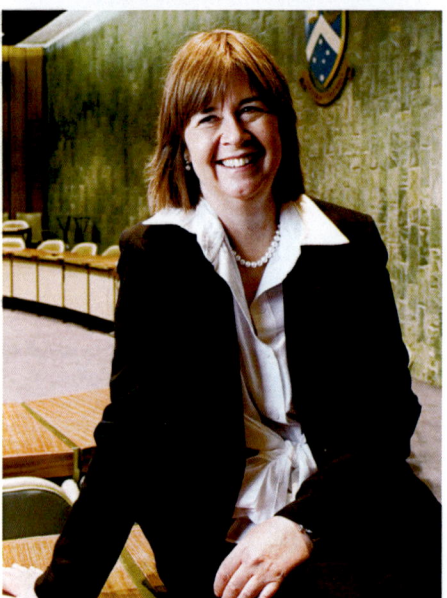

Top left: **Mr Peter Marshall, vice-president (administration), Monash.**

Photographer: Greg Ford.
Courtesy of Monash University.

Top right: **Mr David Pitt, vice-president (finance), Monash.**

Photographer: Greg Ford.
Courtesy of Monash University.

Left: **Professor Edwina Cornish, deputy vice-chancellor and vice-president (research), Monash, 2008.**

Photographer: Andrew Curtis.
Monash University Archives IN7466.

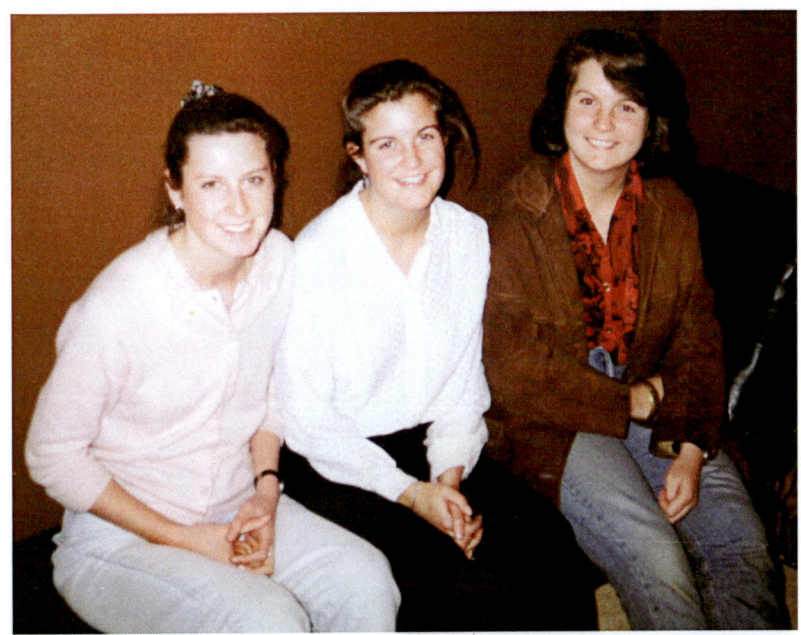

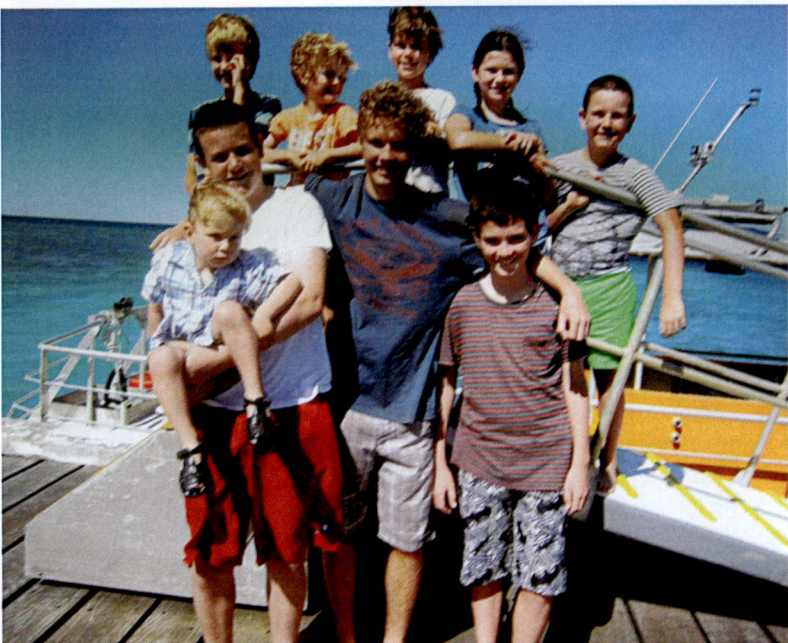

Top: **My daughters (left to right), Kate, Fiona and Sarah, about 1994.**

Above: **Grandchildren, 2014.**

Back row (l–r): Tom, Jasper, Harry, Lucy, Nick. Front row (l–r): Jack holding Finn, Sam, Max.

Both photos from the author's personal collection.

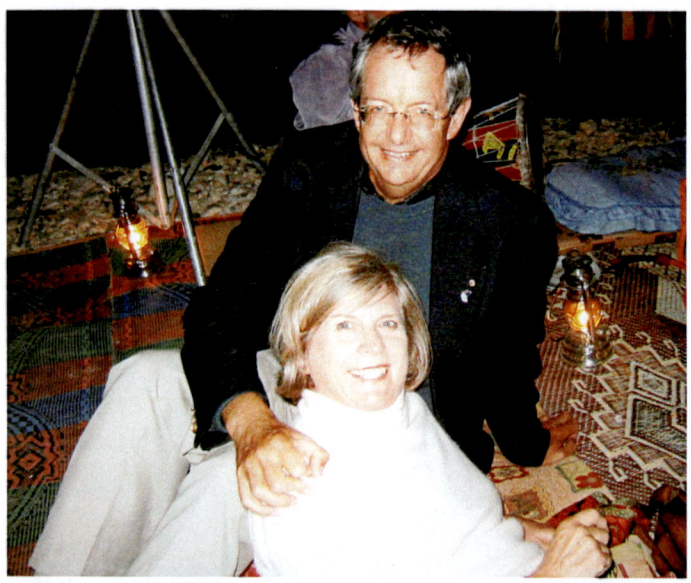

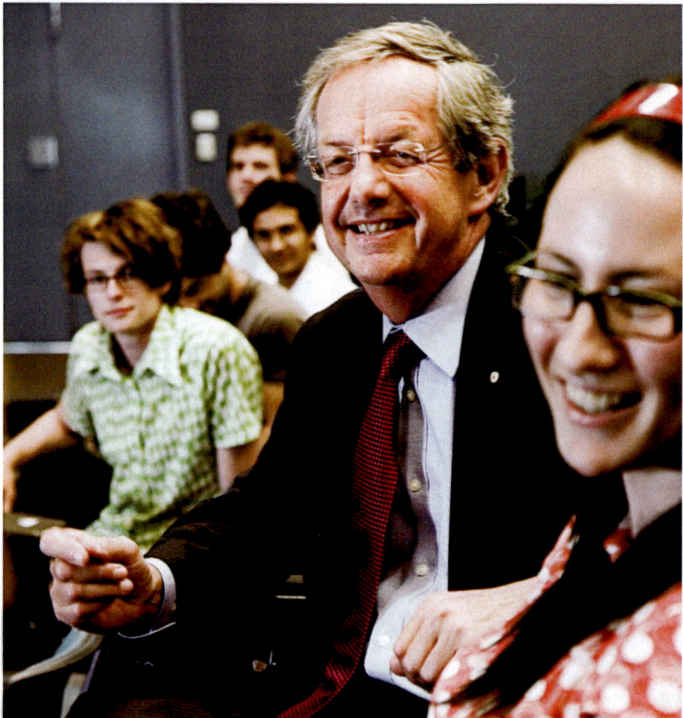

Top: **Celebrating my sixty-third birthday in a Bedouin tent in the Negev Desert, Israel.**
Personal collection.

Above: **With final year medical students in 2008.**
Photographer: Andrew Curtis. Monash University Archives, IN7457.

CHAPTER 17

elderly, who are often on multiple medications for problems in more than one system.

Another issue faced by all the medical colleges was the maintenance of professional standards. It is very obvious that with such rapid advances in the sciences underlying medical practice and with so many new treatments available, it is essential that all doctors continually take active steps to update their knowledge. There are clearly many mechanisms to do this. In my own role as a clinical academic, my involvement in undergraduate education and postgraduate training ensued that I prepared myself by reading relevant literature, speaking to colleagues and learning from my students. Being asked questions that you should know how to answer but find you cannot is a cogent stimulus to continued active learning. But isolated doctors working, for example, in rural environments may not find it so easy not only to be updated, but to realise when they needed to be. Moreover, stories abounded in the media about medical mishaps of one sort or another, where incompetence of the doctor was to blame. This led to pressure for a recertification system. There were strident and zealous advocates of a rigid system that required all doctors to demonstrate that they had fulfilled some defined minimum number of hours of continuing medical education (CME) each year.

I passionately believed that all doctors should be actively involved in CME. However, I was against a mandatory points system. Despite attempts to make it flexible, no such system could account for the learning practices of all doctors. It also encouraged a 'lowest common denominator' approach. There is no arbitrarily defined amount of time spent in CME which is optimal. Most doctors were already conscientious about keeping up to date by one means or another. The points system, which was in wide use, encouraged those who were not conscientious to 'game' the system. They could turn up at the first day of a conference, get their certificate of attendance and not attend any of the serious sessions: CME points and tax deduction in one! It would also lead to a proliferation of low quality educational meetings in exotic places offering CME points.

There is little evidence that mandatory requirements to satisfy minimum quantities of CME is more effective in improving medical practice compared with a voluntary system in which high quality CME material and opportunities are provided under the guidance of the college or similar bodies.

The college had established a Maintenance of Professional Standards program under the sterling leadership of Professor Nick Saunders. This was not mandatory, but was strongly encouraged. Audit of practice was established as an alternative. Over time, with the move to national registration, involvement in an accredited CME program has become mandatory. I maintain my view that it infantilises the profession. Doing something because you have to rather than because you choose to has the risk of taking away motivation from the committed and doing little to convert the uncommitted.

Overall, my involvement with the College of Physicians has been very rewarding. I have become friends with like-minded doctors all over Australia and indeed the English-speaking world. I have learnt a great deal about medicine, the bureaucracy and advocacy.

Chapter 18

APPOINTMENT AT MONASH UNIVERSITY

To my great surprise, towards the end of 2002, the vice-chancellor of the University of Melbourne, Alan Gilbert, asked me whether I would consider becoming the senior deputy vice-chancellor of the university. The incumbent, Professor Sally Walker, had been appointed as the vice-chancellor of Deakin University.

The offer from Alan Gilbert came as a surprise, because although I had enormous personal respect for Alan, I had on many occasions come into conflict about directions in which he was taking the university. I had openly questioned the philosophy of Melbourne University Private and U21 Global, and I had changed the concept and direction of Bio 21. As the dean of the Faculty of Medicine, Dentistry and Health Sciences, there were many instances in which I had to stand up for the faculty against the vice-chancellor and the other faculties. Given the size and budget of our faculty, I had on a number of occasions won the arguments but without endearing our faculty to the rest of the university.

I told Alan that I would consider his offer over the Christmas break. Clearly, it would be a stimulating and exciting position as the second in charge of a large and successful university. It would be interesting and challenging to have to understand the way in which the other faculties worked and to participate in strategies to enhance teaching and research across the whole university. Although it was not an important issue for me, the salary would be significantly greater than I was currently receiving.

The role of the senior deputy vice-chancellor was becoming more and more like that of the provost in the North American system. In universities in the USA, and to a lesser extent Canada, the president (equivalent to our vice-chancellor) was expected to devote more and more of his or her time to advocacy, fundraising and political engagement rather than to the internal affairs of the university. In the case of Alan Gilbert and the University of Melbourne, a significant proportion of Alan's time was taken up with U21 Global and Melbourne University Private, and the senior deputy vice-chancellor was expected to take care of much of the internal affairs of the university, although not with the clearly defined delegation exhibited in the North American system. For example, the deans continued to report to the vice-chancellor. Although Alan had started to expect Sally Walker to share this responsibility, the transition was by no means complete.

After giving the offer considerable thought, I told Alan that although I was very flattered and tempted by the offer, I would respectfully decline it. I was enjoying my role as dean and, at that stage of my career, did not feel inclined to leave a position where I was in charge of the largest faculty in the university, and heavily involved and influential in the health sector in general, to become second in charge of the university. It sounds arrogant as I recount it, and I am sure it sounded arrogant to Alan, but it was a true reflection of how I felt. He took it graciously. A number of months later, Alan was appointed as the vice-chancellor of the University of Manchester, which was undertaking an amalgamation with the Manchester Institute of Science and Technology, a position he held with distinction until his untimely death in 2009. It is possible that Alan was trying to position me so I was well-placed to succeed him at the University of Melbourne. If this is so, he did not hint at it. Even if I had been in that position, there is obviously no certainty that I would subsequently have been appointed vice-chancellor. And in any case, for me, the role I undertook at Monash was more appealing. I had been at the University of Melbourne for most of my academic life and a completely new challenge at a different university was more exciting, despite the prestige of the University of Melbourne.

Until Alan approached me about the senior deputy vice-chancellor appointment at the University of Melbourne, I had not seriously contemplated becoming a vice-chancellor. I was almost sixty, I had always been deeply immersed in medicine and other areas of health and was very happy at the prospect of continuing in my role of dean for a further three years or so and then to continue or expand clinical practice and maybe resume my research. But Alan Gilbert's approach started me thinking about the role. I did not want to be second in charge, but maybe if in some unlikely circumstance I had the opportunity, it could be a new and interesting challenge to lead

CHAPTER 18

a university. I was totally committed to the broad role of universities in education and research and considered them vital to the future, not only of Australia, but of the planet.

It occurred to me that Monash University must be some way along the process of appointing a new vice-chancellor. David Robinson had been forced to resign around the middle of 2002, following a widely publicised scandal relating to alleged plagiarism. The episode reflected a sharply divided university. Robinson had been regarded by many as autocratic, with a number of the usual moderating structures of the university, such as the academic board, effectively bypassed during his tenure. The committee of deans was his sounding-board, but this did not lead to effective communication with the university as a whole. Moreover, Robinson's imaginative, indeed visionary, international plans were at best controversial, with many of the academic staff feeling they were unrealistic and would prevent the university from performing competitively in research. This particularly applied to the South African campus, which was clearly struggling to attract students and performing well behind budget and costing the university a lot of money. To compound the problems, the disruptions and unrest caused by the amalgamations of the early 1990s had not yet subsided, leading to further restlessness and dissatisfaction amongst the academic and general staff of the university.

A strong body of the senior academic staff felt that David Robinson's leadership was flawed both in style and content. Eagle-eyed academic colleagues trawling over Robinson's publications came upon a book on alcoholism written and published in the 1970s, in which a section of text closely resembled text from another source. It was not footnoted or referenced, although the source was listed in the bibliography of the book, hardly a strategy that someone who had knowingly and wilfully plagiarised an academic work would employ. Robinson argued that this was the result of carelessness and not misconduct, but the publicity, first apparent in the *Sunday Times* in the UK, forced his resignation.

The deputy vice-chancellor (research), Peter Darvall, was appointed as the vice-chancellor for the period before the formal process of seeking and appointing a new vice-chancellor could be completed. Peter had been a member of the academic staff of Monash University since 1970. He had held many appointments, including professor of civil engineering and dean of the Faculty of Engineering before his appointment as deputy vice-chancellor (research) in 1993, a position he held until his appointment as vice-chancellor and president on Robinson's resignation. He knew Monash backwards, he was an engaging speaker and had enough of the rogue in him to appeal to the younger sibling character of Monash in contrast with the more established and traditional character of the University of Melbourne. Darvall had shown outstanding leadership in the aftermath of a tragic incident at Monash late in 2002, when a deranged student had shot and killed two students in a postgraduate economics class and injured others. The incident had severely traumatised the university and Darvall's leadership during this time was faultless.

I had no idea how far the definitive process of appointing the new vice-chancellor had progressed or indeed whether the process would be bypassed and Peter Darvall asked to continue in the role he was obviously filling very well.

I looked up the internet and found that the position had been advertised three months earlier. I assumed that the process would be too far advanced for there to be any interest in me, but I thought nothing would be lost by a phone call. Interested potential applicants had been invited to contact David Pumphrey from the search company Heidrick and Struggles. I was not sure whether I had been transported back to the London of Charles Dickens, but I phoned David. He was a charming man who I got to know quite well over the ensuing couple of weeks. I said who I was and gave him my background. I said also that I assumed I was too late, and in any case, they probably had no interest in a dean of medicine – if they did, they had an outstanding one in Nick Saunders at Monash. He said that the interviews with shortlisted candidates were to take place in ten days, but he would speak to the chancellor, Jerry Ellis, to see if he had any interest.

David phoned me shortly after and said that Jerry would be interested to meet me and could I have dinner with him at a restaurant in the city. I did so and we spent a fair bit of time talking about a mutual passion we had for golf. Jerry was obviously impressed that I had been invited to be president of the Royal Melbourne Golf Club. Of course, we also discussed the university, what I had done in the past and why I was interested.

I spoke to my long-standing friend and colleague, Nick Saunders, who was dean of the Faculty of Medicine, Nursing and Health Sciences at Monash and who I thought would be a very strong candidate for the position of vice-chancellor. He indicated that he was not in a position to take up such a post

CHAPTER 18

and indeed intended to retire as dean and return to Newcastle for pressing family reasons. He was very supportive of my application.

In the event, I was invited to submit a vision statement and curriculum vitae and to take part in the final selection process. This turned out to be quite an experience in its own right. The council had been persuaded that in order to ensure that the university as a whole had a real role in the appointment of the new vice-chancellor, the shortlisted candidates would be interviewed for an hour by each of four panels made up of university academic and general staff and students. The panels each covered a separate area – education, research, finances and management. Following this, there was a one-and-a-half-hour interview with the selection committee itself. The panels would provide input to the selection committee, and the selection committee, which was chaired by the chancellor, Jerry Ellis, would then make a recommendation to council.

Before the interview, I phoned David Robinson and asked whether he would be prepared to see me. Graciously, he agreed to do so. Although obviously scarred by the process, he gave a lot of background about Monash and was very encouraging.

Although tiring, I enjoyed the process of interviews by the panels followed by the selection committee. I had nothing to lose. I was perfectly happy in my current role and my career goals, to the extent I had identified them, had not included being a vice-chancellor. The preliminary discussions with the panels better prepared my thoughts for the definitive interview with the selection committee.

I was told that four candidates had been shortlisted for interview. The interviews were conducted in the Monash city building at 30 Collins Street. In order to keep the candidates apart and the process confidential, rooms in the Sofitel Hotel across Collins Street were used as staging posts for the candidates, and each was assigned a minder from the human resources staff. Given their elaborate security preparations, it was unfortunate that when I was escorted into a lift at the Sofitel a long-time research colleague from interstate was in the lift, also accompanied by a minder. It was obvious why we were both there, so we greeted each other warmly and with a certain degree of amusement, to the embarrassment of our respective minders.

The interview went smoothly enough but with no indication of whether I was really hitting the mark with my responses. I took-off the next day for Hong Kong, where I was to join a panel reviewing medical education in

Hong Kong for the local medical registration authority. Not too long after my arrival, I received a phone call from the chancellor to say that I was very much under consideration but that there was a process to go through. He expressed a certain amount of frustration with the academic process and said that in business it was the outcome that mattered, but that academics seemed to be overly concerned about process. I heard nothing more for a number of days and proceeded with what turned out to be a most intriguing week in Hong Kong.

When we visited the Chinese University of Hong Kong's teaching hospital in Shatin, we were told that a most unusual form of influenza or some similar illness had struck the hospital, with a significant number of medical and nursing staff affected and off duty. It turned out that this was the first manifestation in Hong Kong of SARS (severe acute respiratory syndrome), a newly emergent disease with a high fatality rate. It rapidly became headlines around the world.

The director of health in Hong Kong, Margaret Chan, entertained the panel for dinner during the week. She spoke extensively of the new infection that was causing such a problem in Hong Kong and steps she was taking to identify the causative agent and to control its spread. At that time, it seemed that it might well cause a lethal world pandemic, wreaking havoc like the Spanish influenza epidemic of 1918–19. Margaret Chan was later criticised quite strongly by the Legislative Council in Hong Kong for not acting quickly or decisively enough, although later still it was realised that lack of information from the Chinese mainland had prevented a more vigorous approach.

In the event, the epidemic was controlled and largely confined to mainland China, Hong Kong and Singapore, with some cases in North America. One of our panel, the head of the Hong Kong Hospital Authority, contracted SARS. Thankfully, he survived. Margaret Chan's career was not permanently harmed, as she was appointed director general of the World Health Organisation in 2006.

Being in the centre of what at the time seemed as though it might be the start of the anticipated and feared global pandemic of an emergent disease thousands of kilometres from Melbourne was a sufficient distraction from the machinations of the appointment process. Eventually, after returning from Hong Kong, I was told I was the preferred candidate and that my

CHAPTER 18

name would be recommended to council, who would have to endorse the recommendation.

On the Saturday morning following my return from Hong Kong, I received a phone call from Peter Darvall congratulating me on my appointment. This seemed strange, as council had not met and the appointment would depend on its endorsement. Peter said that it was in the *Australian*.

I duly obtained a copy and saw that the newspaper had announced my appointment, albeit prematurely, with the far from encouraging headline, 'Outside Appointment Divides a Fractured University'. There had obviously been a leak from the appointment committee. There was reference to the committee being evenly divided between me and an internal candidate, with the chancellor's will eventually holding sway. I had no idea if this was so and no interest in knowing who was supporting me and who was supporting the internal candidate, who turned out to be the dean of law, Stephen Parker.

I did know that Stephen was a highly intelligent individual with a strong strategic bent, who had been a prominent figure in the university, including as the author, with the pro vice-chancellor (planning and quality), Graham Webb, of the document 'Leading the Way', in 2002. This document was to provide the blueprint for the direction of Monash over the next few years. Thus, it would have been strange if he did not have strong internal support, particularly given my background, which was closely identified with the University of Melbourne and also my medical background. The discipline of medicine is always regarded with suspicion by other faculties in universities, particularly by the humanities and social sciences.

If the mode of the premature public announcement of my appointment was inauspicious, so too was the official confirmation of it by the council at the Clayton campus. I was told to come to the front of building 3a and I would be shown where to park. I discovered where the building was and duly arrived in my twelve-year-old Alfa Romeo 75 – my pride and joy, but at that stage distinctly showing its age and behaving even more erratically than had been its wont. After getting instructions from the executive assistant of the council secretary on where to park, I attempted to restart the car. The starting mechanism jammed and I could not budge it. The EA called for help, and a number of her colleagues who were the executive support of the senior staff of the university came and pushed my car out of the way. This was their introduction to the person who was meant to lead Monash to a better place!

I then waited outside while the council debated the confirmation of my appointment. After what seemed like an inordinate time, the chancellor came out and said that the council had decided to offer me the position. I indicated my acceptance in principle, and we all had a drink together.

I wanted to round off things at the University of Melbourne and also to have some time off before starting, so I negotiated a starting date of 1 September 2003, some five months after the appointment.

Back at the University of Melbourne, my acceptance of the position was taken by some as being foolhardy ('nothing and no one could save Monash') or as betrayal. In the latter category was my executive assistant for the last nineteen years, Liz Mobilio. Liz had been a very loyal and efficient assistant to me, first in my role as the James Stewart Professor of Medicine at the Royal Melbourne Hospital and then in my time as dean. She had started working for me as a relatively inexperienced person in her early twenties and had developed into a highly intelligent and competent executive assistant. During that time, she had completed a BA degree part-time. It was a difficult decision not to suggest that she come with me to Monash, but I felt that I needed someone who knew Monash well and could help me to gain the confidence of the Monash community. I am pleased to say that after some difficult times, Liz has for some time been the executive assistant to the deputy vice-chancellor (global engagement) at the University of Melbourne, Susan Elliott, a survivor and major contributor to the introduction of the new medical school curriculum in 1999.

One of the most difficult aspects of the new position was the necessity to give up my medical practice. Although my involvement with the Royal Melbourne Hospital had decreased substantially when I became dean, so that I was only occasionally able to attend endocrinology outpatients, I had managed to maintain a half day per week of private practice. I had been managing the diabetes, thyroid, pituitary or other endocrine diseases of many of these patients for up to twenty-five years, and they had loyally followed me through a variety of second-rate consulting rooms at the Repat and in corners of the Department of Medicine at the Royal Melbourne before finally arriving at reasonably professional quarters in the private wing of the hospital. I was still being referred interesting patients and enjoyed the opportunity to be a proper doctor at least for a small part of each week.

CHAPTER 18

So it was sad to stop doing the only thing I had been trained to do and to say goodbye to my patients, some of whom I had seen from adolescence, through marriage and childbirth and divorce. I arranged their transfer and they seemed to understand, but it did make me sad.

Still, a new challenge and a new opportunity beckoned and I was grateful to have the opportunity of what was, in many senses, a new career just as I was turning sixty. An old dog and a new trick!

Chapter 19

EARLY DAYS AT MONASH UNIVERSITY

Like most people appointed to leadership positions at new organisations, I had resolved to spend most of the first three months speaking to people and learning about the university before making any significant decisions. I soon discovered that this was a luxury I could not afford and in any case it was somewhat foreign to my natural inclination to say what I think when the opportunity arises.

There had been some significant interactions even before I took up the position, where I had to make important decisions or to at least declare my hand.

The first related to Stephen Parker. It was now common knowledge that Stephen was the internal candidate who had narrowly failed to be appointed. He was very well respected in the university. Peter Marshall, then the director of human resources, phoned me to say that Stephen was considering leaving and taking up a deputy vice-chancellor position at another Group of Eight university. Peter advised me that this would be a pity, as Stephen had much to offer and would be a big loss to the university. I met with Stephen, discussed the situation and advised the council to offer Stephen the position of deputy vice-chancellor (academic). Stephen eventually accepted this appointment and was later appointed as the senior deputy vice-chancellor.

Stephen was a major contributor during our time working together at Monash. He was highly strategic, but also very organised. He was responsible for bringing together many of the planning documents for the university. We were in many ways complementary. My style was informal and I was intent on building the morale and self-esteem of the university, which had been severely battered by recent events. Stephen was much

CHAPTER 19

more disciplined and formal in his approach and was often frustrated by my informality. I remain grateful for his very considerable contribution to Monash's resurgence during the time we worked together. He is now a vigorous and reforming vice-chancellor of the University of Canberra. Despite tensions which emerged from time to time, I think my decision to keep Stephen at Monash, at least for a time, was the correct one for Monash.

The next time it was necessary for me to declare my hand even before taking up the appointment was at an off-site senior management planning meeting convened by Peter Darvall. The introductory comments at the meeting were along the lines that Monash University could not hope to compete with the University of Melbourne because of some inherent disadvantages. The first was that it was twenty kilometres from the CBD. The second was that as a result of the Dawkins 'Reforms' of the late 1980s and early 1990s, it had been lumbered with a regional campus (Gippsland) and two outer suburban campuses (Peninsula and Berwick). Along with the Caulfield campus, these campuses had not been research-intensive and would dilute both the research effort and the reputation of the university and therefore its ability to attract top students to it. There was also criticism of the international strategy and the impact that was having on the finances available to support research in Australia and on management time and effort.

I felt it necessary at that time to put in a contrary argument. I felt that the location of the Clayton campus was actually a comparative advantage compared with the University of Melbourne. It was in the middle of the major centre for manufacturing in Victoria (apart from the main automotive manufacturing plants), collocated with the largest research campus of CSIRO and with sufficient space around it to be chosen as the site of the proposed Australian synchrotron. In contrast, the University of Melbourne was landlocked, surrounded by extremely expensive real estate and very active local government planning controls, together with a vocal local residents association.

The University of Melbourne had also felt extremely vulnerable in the political sense because it did not have a general campus in a regional location. At the same time, it was trying to offload or close some of the agricultural colleges it had acquired in the mergers of the Dawkins era, which had small and diminishing numbers of students and were clearly non-viable. This sense of vulnerability had led the vice-chancellor Alan Gilbert to declare Shepparton, to its surprise, a University of Melbourne town at the time the Rural Clinical School was opened there. The Gippsland campus was a political asset and also served a real need in providing tertiary educational opportunity to rural students not otherwise able to access universities. Berwick and Peninsula could not hope to emulate Clayton, but each could develop areas of strength with research excellence in special areas of local relevance.

The international strategy was imaginative and bold. It would distinguish Monash and prevent it becoming a grey shadow of Melbourne.

Finally, I felt compelled to say that if Monash regarded Melbourne as its main competitor, it had lost sight of the main game. Monash was out to be the very best university it could be in an absolute sense. If there were competitors, these were spread around the globe. We would be a more effective university in every sense if we could collaborate constructively with the University of Melbourne, other Australian universities and like-minded universities around the world.

The third significant interaction I had before starting formally at Monash was with the Monash Student Association (MSA). I received an email from the president of MSA inviting me to meet with her executive committee. The president, Shen, was a law student. The student associations of the various campuses had not amalgamated with the mergers and in the best traditions of the old Monash the Clayton MSA was very left-wing. In contrast, the Student Union at Caulfield was a right-wing organisation and fiercely opposed to the MSA at Clayton.

Of course, I accepted the invitation to meet with the MSA, which I did in their home territory in the Campus Centre at Monash, Clayton. I was confronted with T-shirts with slogans such as 'the Monash Sausage Factory' and 'Robinson, President of the Monash Corporation'.

I was asked, somewhat aggressively, what I thought a university should do and be. I answered honestly, with my views about the role of universities in educating the leaders of the future, in providing life-transforming opportunities for all and in advancing knowledge for the betterment of humankind. They seemed a little taken aback and said that that was their idea of a university too. I replied that they would then understand that if I did things they did not like, it was because I was acting under constraints that they did not have. If that occurred, they should come and speak with

CHAPTER 19

me, and I would explain the constraints I was facing. I would then give them the opportunity of explaining how they would act in the face of the constraints, given that we now knew we were aiming for the same outcomes.

I was at first gratified and then apprehensive to receive a Christmas card from Shen at the end of 2003, three months after starting as vice-chancellor stating: 'Dear Richard, we think you are a good man in the true sense of the word, so remember that next year when the trouble starts'. I could not claim months later that I had not been warned!

After moving farewells from the Faculty of Medicine, Dentistry and Health Sciences and from the vice-chancellor, the senior executive group and my fellow deans at the University of Melbourne, and following a brief break overseas, I finally started at Monash University on 1 September 2003.

It was clear from my first day that the university was deeply divided. The senior management team, or Vice-Chancellor's Group (VCG) as it was known, comprised individuals who had been strong supporters of David Robinson and his policies and those who were deeply opposed to him. The first meetings of this group were tense, with the combined suspicion of me coming in as an outsider and of each other. The individuals involved were all people of talent and experience, but the net effect was dysfunctional. I soon came to the conclusion that it would be necessary to make some changes, but I could not afford to do this precipitously. This would have had the combined effect of heightening tensions, increasing the difficulties I faced as an outsider and losing a considerable amount of talent. Moreover, given the contractual situation, it was impractical to make abrupt changes without huge expense to the university. Instead, supported by the chancellor, I made gradual changes, some of which were achieved by encouraging members of the team to pursue new opportunities elsewhere and others by not renewing contracts when they were due or prematurely terminating contracts. In each case, the ends were achieved by negotiation and each person was given a 'soft landing', with a genuine acknowledgement of all their contributions to Monash. After two years, it was a very different VCG, and by four years, there had been a complete turnover of each position. At the end of my time, we had a highly effective and collegial VCG, to my mind at least the equal of any university in Australia.

A lot of water was to flow under the bridge before that.

On my first day at Monash, I addressed an open forum of staff members. Several hundred came to the Alexandra Theatre. I tried then to be brief and informal rather than to deliver a treatise on my theories of tertiary education. I emphasised the enthusiasm I had for the position, my view that Monash University had achieved an incredible amount in a short time and that through its trajectory and international positioning was best placed of any Australian university to become a truly great university on the global scale. I emphasised my total commitment to the highest quality of education and research as being fundamental to achieving this outcome and my view that the importance of doing so was not for the glory of Monash, but because the world needed great universities to educate the leaders of the future and to solve the environmental, energy, food security, health, poverty, trade, governance and legal challenges facing the world. Although achieving adequate funding was essential to accomplishing these objectives, this was a means to an end, not an end in its own right. To allay concerns that the university had become too corporate under David Robinson, I either reassured the audience or alarmed them by pointing out that my approach was the antithesis of the corporate model. This address seemed to be well received.

As with any change of leadership in a large organisation, there was an opportunity for the university to reassess where it was and where it wanted to go. I suggested that we have a planning conference comprising VCG, the deans, heads of campuses, heads of schools and departments and the senior non-academic administrative staff. It was held off-site in the Yarra Valley some five months after I started. I presented my appraisal of where Monash stood in its quest to become a world-class university and called my talk 'A Glass Half Full'. I summarised my view of the outstanding achievements of Monash to date and the unresolved problems and challenges it faced.

I presented a strategic framework stating the major steps we needed to take and the strategies needed to achieve these. It built on the 'Leading the Way Document' written in 2002 by Stephen Parker and Graham Webb, the pro vice-chancellor (planning and quality), and it listed a set of guiding values for the university. These had been extensively 'workshopped' through VCG and the committee of deans. I emphasised that the value dealing with self-reliance was at the end of the list. It was essential that we work towards this, but we should always remember that this was to enable the university

CHAPTER 19

to achieve its higher order objectives in education, research and external engagement.

I was delighted when the conference endorsed, apparently with enthusiasm, a new statement of purpose (mission statement) for the university. 'Monash University seeks to improve the human condition and foster creativity. It does so through research and education and a commitment to human rights, social justice and a sustainable environment.' A little soft and fuzzy, perhaps, but we all seemed to think it was what Monash is about.

We had an external consultant address us about external perceptions of Monash and challenges it faced. David Phillips had an extensive background in the federal education bureaucracy and in recent years had earned a high reputation as a consultant on higher education. He used the metaphor of a large rowing boat. The challenge for Monash was not so much to get everyone rowing in time, but to have them rowing in vaguely the same direction. He also highlighted challenges ahead with moves to partially deregulate the undergraduate student contribution to their tuition fees (HECS), a likely greater contest for and perhaps reduced number of international students and the increasing importance of international ranking systems for universities.

Overall, the conference had a very positive and optimistic feel about it. The university knew that it faced challenges and needed to resolve some issues about which there were no common views. But it also knew by the end of the conference that the highest priority was to be placed on the educational and research performance of the university and that the academic staff would be fully supported to achieve this. Excellence in education and research were to be valued equally highly – they were the twin peaks that good universities must climb. They were interdependent and fed off each other. Monash must and could improve its performance in both.

In terms of unresolved issues, the multi-campus domestic structure and the international strategy were those which attracted the most controversy, and each will be dealt with in some detail. But first, the management and financial structures and systems needed to be addressed to ensure that there was an effective process to enable them to serve the higher order objectives of the university in education and research. As I often pointed out during my time at Monash, we could have the best educators and researchers in the world, but we would be a total disaster as an institution if we did not have appropriate administrative and financial structures with the necessary expertise to guide them.

An early challenge that confronted me was an exciting but foundering initiative that David Robinson and the then dean of the Faculty of Information Technology, John Rosenberg, had initiated for Monash. This was a joint initiative with the International Olympic Committee (IOC) to manage the knowledge gained at each Olympic Games and to pass it on to the next local organising committee. It would also involve educational programs for Olympic officials. There was a local joint venture company involving Monash with a board including representatives from Rino and Lorenz Grollo's Equiset company and other private interests and an international governing committee with representatives of the IOC, including Kevan Gosper, vice-president of the IOC. It was a novel and exciting venture, but it had come off the rails. Management of the Australian joint venture company was less than ideal, Monash was not well equipped to deal with the data management task, and the relations between the deputy vice-chancellor Alison Crook and some of the external board members had soured. But from my point of view, the overarching problem was that the agreement with the IOC had been set up in such a way that Monash was required to invest its resources, both real and in kind, but any profits or dividends from the activity would be returned to the IOC and not to Monash.

When I inherited this situation and after discussion with the key participants, I decided that it was in the interests of Monash to withdraw from the project. Monash had already invested AUS$1.5 million in the enterprise as well as considerable time and effort, and further investment seemed to me to be futile with no potential upside. Moreover, there was considerable reputation risk for Monash, particularly given the less-than-satisfactory progress so far made in the task of data management and the relatively disorganised state of the joint venture company.

I was due to go the USA to a meeting between the Group of Eight university vice-chancellors (Melbourne, Monash, Sydney, New South Wales, Australian National University, Queensland, Adelaide and Western Australia) and our counterparts from the sixty leading research universities in the United States. Following that meeting, I was planning to go to Europe to visit our London Centre, to meet with the University of Leiden about a possible partnership and to visit our Prato Centre. I decided that it would be best to meet directly with the IOC in Lausanne as well. This

CHAPTER 19

trip in total occupied just over a week and set the tone for a number of exhausting overseas visits to Monash's far-flung campuses and centres and for graduations, alumni events and to meet potential partners.

In Lausanne, I met with the president of the IOC, Jacques Rogge. He was formal but friendly and when I explained Monash's position and my responsibility for its financial performance, he agreed to purchase Monash's shares in the business. We therefore recovered about AUS$800,000 of the AUS$1,500,000 that had been invested to date. Importantly, we parted with good relations apparently maintained and with an expressed willingness of the IOC to call on Monash on a contract basis whenever it seemed appropriate. I am not sure that it ever has, but to me the important thing was that we had extracted ourselves from a situation that was potentially going to cost us a lot of money and which held considerable reputational risk. I regarded it as an important lesson in how careful universities must be in taking on projects outside their core mission in research and education.

After the negotiations were completed, Kevan Gosper entertained us at a fine dinner, indicating that there were no hard feelings on behalf of the IOC. Gosper and the Grollos handled the potentially awkward situation impeccably and with great integrity.

Chapter 20

THE END OF THE HONEYMOON – STUDENT RIOTS AND A FLASHBACK TO THE 1960s

University funding had been progressively decreased in real terms following the election of the Howard conservative government in 1996. The term 'Vanstone cuts' had become part of the lexicon on university campuses as shorthand for the savage reduction in funding imposed by the minister for education, Senator Amanda Vanstone. They were part of a general policy of cutting government expenditure to balance the budget and to reduce the government debt inherited by the Howard government. To those of us who saw education and research as fundamental to the future economic prosperity and wellbeing of the nation, the cuts to public expenditure on universities appeared short-sighted and counterproductive.

Brendan Nelson was the minister for education when I took up my position, and he had instituted a review of university funding. This resulted in a number of changes, known collectively as the 'Nelson Reforms'. The most radical and significant of these from the point of view of the universities was partial deregulation of the student contribution to the cost of their education through the Higher Education Contribution Scheme or HECS.

Introduced by the Hawke-Keating Labor government in 1989 as part of the Dawkins reforms, the HECS was an innovative scheme to share the cost of university education between the government and the student in recognition that there was both public and private benefit from higher education. The novel aspects of the scheme which was devised by economist Bruce Chapman were that there was no requirement for up-front contributions, no interest charged on the 'loan' and repayment was deferred until the income of the graduate was above a certain threshold,

CHAPTER 20

approximating the average income for working Australians. There was then a graduated repayment depending on income added to the tax payable by the individual. The student or their family could choose to pay the fees 'upfront' with a discount of about 25 per cent.

This elegant scheme meant that students from economically disadvantaged backgrounds could access higher education with no need for upfront fees. If their income never rose to a reasonable level, there was no need for repayment, and even when it did rise to levels above the average income, the repayment schedule was relatively painless, as it was automatically added to the tax rate at manageable levels. The scheme has been adopted in other countries, reflecting that it is the fairest way to share the contributions to the cost of higher education between the state and the individual, recognising benefits to both. Of course, once introduced, there will always be a temptation by governments to increase the student contributions. This had happened at the time of the 'Vanstone cuts', where not only had the HECS rate increased, but differential rates for different disciplines reflecting perceived differences in public benefit and potential individual remuneration in the different disciplines had been introduced. These rates were still set by government, with no flexibility for different institutions to set different HECS rates.

The changes introduced by Brendan Nelson included the right of universities to set their own HECS rates from zero up to a maximum of 25 per cent above the standard rate. The idea was to introduce competition and to allow universities to increase their income without any increase in the cost to government.

Students vigorously opposed any increase to the student contribution through increased HECS. On the other hand, cash-strapped universities felt that there was no alternative but to increase the HECS fee to the maximum allowed if they were to maintain standards. Most moved to do this in the first year of the new legislation and those that did not followed within the next year or so.

The Monash Student Association at Clayton fiercely opposed the increase and started a vigorous campaign. On the day that council was meeting to debate and presumably agree to increase the HECS contribution by the maximum allowable 25 per cent, the MSA had arranged a substantial protest, which included an attempted invasion of the council chamber in the centre of the main administration building. They gained entrance through Robert Blackwood Hall and stampeded along the ceremonial walkway using the ends of fire hoses to knock down doors. Security guards were trampled. The council was rapidly evacuated through a back entrance of the administration building and relocated secretly to the facilities building on a separate part of the campus. The motion to increase the HECS contribution by 25 per cent was passed.

The protest gained considerable media publicity. The MSA, led by the formidable Shen, had used the old trick of setting off fire alarms in the Menzies building, placed some placard-wielding students in the midst of the throng of evacuated staff and students and arranged for television cameras to film the apparent large protests. Shen announced that there would be another protest in two days' time.

Given the damage to property and the injury to security staff, I saw no alternative but to ask for a police presence during the proposed subsequent protest. I asked to meet with Shen. I explained the rationale for the decision by council and also indicated that because of the damage to property and individuals during the first protest, the police would be on site during their proposed protest the next day. We had no objection to peaceful protest, but the police had indicated that if they came, we had to understand that they would arrest people who broke the law, so she and her colleagues should be careful. The discussions had been cordial and respectful.

The next morning, Shen appeared on John Faine's morning radio show on ABC Radio claiming that the vice-chancellor had threatened her with arrest despite the fact that they only wished to have a peaceful protest.

The demonstration duly proceeded. Two hundred or more students occupied the old vice-chancellor's residence, then used as the headquarters of marketing and public affairs. They invited me to come and meet with them. Always believing that logical discussion with reasonable people can resolve most issues, I agreed to come and meet them. Stephen Parker came with me but was wise enough to stay silent.

I was confronted by an unruly mob of students and ex-students. I started to explain the rationale for the increase in HECS fees. I was interrupted by abusive rants. I said that I had not come to be vilified and abused and would leave if this continued. The students then had a vote and, by a narrow margin, vilification and abuse were ruled out of order. Six or so of the students had orange sashes around them labelled 'Legal Observers' – presumably they were the law students.

CHAPTER 20

I attempted to explain that the HECS system was an equitable one, as it allowed some payback to the government from those who had benefited from subsidised higher education. No upfront fees were required, so it should not deter those from lower socio-economic groups from coming to university, and it would allow more bursaries to support the living costs of such students. The universities had no choice but to increase the HECS contribution if the quality of the students' educational experience was to be maintained or improved.

At this point, a student with a bandana around his head leapt on to a table and screamed, 'He is a liar and a hypocrite! They are all liars and hypocrites! The revolution has to start here!' At this point, I did not think that anything more could be achieved, so Stephen and I left.

I was severely reprimanded by the police, as they said that I should not have gone into the protest without their permission and without a police escort.

The occupation ended after a couple of days and much noise but little outcome for the students apart from a lot of publicity. Another occupation of the international office a few days later also ended peacefully, although it had a more sinister side, as three staff, including Tony Pollock, the vice-president, international, were held hostage for some hours in rather intimidating circumstances.

Despite my warning, Shen was arrested, allegedly for throwing a rock through a plate glass window and for stealing a policeman's hat. Two other students were arrested, one the Chinese Australian who had leapt on to the top of the table during the occupation in the Che Guevara style and the other a student of middle eastern background.

The protests did have their amusing side, which included posters pasted all over the campus with my photo in Arab headdress and with the caption: 'Osama bin Larkins, Terrorist Against Public Education'.

Overall, I found the protests and their personal nature quite discomforting and I understood how Louis Matheson had felt during the prolonged student unrest during the late 1960s and early 1970s. Although the period of unrest was shorter this time, it was by no means totally benign. There was damage to property and some level of injury and upset to our security staff. As a result of the police action to arrest the main offenders as identified by the police themselves and the fact that they were not of white Caucasian origins, the words 'Racist Scum' were painted on the pavement pointing to my office.

NEW TRICKS

Most of all, I felt somewhat betrayed by the MSA, given my attempts to build good relations with them and the subsequent personal nature of the attacks.

I held a public forum to discuss the issues, attended by quite a number of staff and students. I did my best to answer questions honestly and not to be vindictive. I did point out the need for protests to respect the safety of individuals and the value of property.

Things subsided after that. The HECS increases became universal around Australia.

As a postscript, when Shen's trial finally came to court about twelve months later, she asked me to be a character witness. Despite my disappointment with elements of her behaviour and that of her colleagues, I gave her a positive reference, indicating that although she was headstrong and impulsive, she had strong leadership qualities and would be likely to really make a difference in the future.

She was reprimanded with no conviction recorded – an important outcome, given that she was a law student and a conviction would have impacted on her ability to practise.

At the end of this episode, I felt I had really been blooded as a vice-chancellor.

Chapter 21

ADMINISTRATION AND FINANCE

One of many issues contributing to angst at the university at the time I started was the introduction of a new form of budgeting known as strategic cost management or SCM. Alison Crook, the innovative deputy vice-chancellor of resources, was responsible for introducing it. It depended on using the capacity of the financial systems to analyse costs according to the activities in the university and then assigning them to the various faculties or centres according to the extent to which they contributed to or utilised the identified activities. The real costs of occupying space was included in this analysis and categorised according to whether the space was considered high cost, moderate or low cost in terms of building it and fitting it out and in terms of the costs of maintaining it.

Similarly, sources of income were related to the activities earning the income and the faculty or centre responsible for doing so.

This type of analysis revealed that by looking at the income and costs associated with various activities, some parts of the university were running at a considerable loss, whereas others were generating financial surpluses. Moreover, some types of activities were consistently losing money, whereas others were making money for the university. For example, conducting laboratory-based research, taking on Australian PhD students, performance studies in music and theatre and studio-based fine arts studies were all losing considerable money. In contrast, teaching international students in undergraduate courses such as business, accounting and law generated significant surpluses.

The 'strategic' part of SCM then meant that the university had to decide which of the activities that were losing money were important strategically to the university and working out how these could be reconfigured in a more cost-effective way or, alternatively, cross-subsidised.

The budgeting worked by assigning the income to the academic units which generated it and then charging for all the administrative and support services, including space on the basis of the use of the services or space by the academic units. Each faculty was given a targeted financial outcome which might be a substantial cash surplus to allow it to cross-subsidise other areas which were not operating in surplus.

Monash was the first Australian university to introduce this methodology. It had the great advantage of promoting transparency and incentives for faculties to demand less space and to utilise services in a more considered way. It encouraged them to pursue actively methods to raise revenue. It provided pressure on the administrative service units to cut costs for services, as these were now visible and could be compared with costs charged by commercial suppliers. It allowed rational decisions about 'outsourcing' non-academic activities which were not being provided efficiently internally.

In some situations, the case for cross-subsidisation was clear cut. Research grants from national competitive funding sources such as the Australian Research Council (ARC) and the National Health and Medical Research Council (NHMRC) were highly competitive and prestigious. They came with some accompanying infrastructure funding for the indirect costs of research, but this was insufficient to cover the real costs. It was estimated that the shortfall was about fifty cents for every dollar of research funding attracted. The more successful a faculty or department was, the more difficulty it would have in achieving a balanced budget. Similarly, scholarships for PhD students did not take account of the indirect costs of their research and the additional funding provided to the university was also insufficient to cover these costs fully. If the university really wanted to be a leading research-intensive university, it must ensure that these costs were adequately funded.

The fees (a composite of the student contribution or HECS and the government contribution) for teaching Australian undergraduate students were tightly regulated and had effectively fallen in real terms from the time indexation was replaced by a 'cost adjustment factor' in 1995. The number of students in each discipline was also tightly regulated. The cost adjustment each year was well below the increased costs generated by inflation and even further below the true increase in costs taking into account salary increases and the need for technological upgrading, maintenance of buildings and new buildings to accommodate increased numbers of students. The increased costs

CHAPTER 21

could be accommodated in some cases, where the students mostly attended large lectures such as in law, business and economics and the humanities, although even in these areas, there had to be associated increases in sizes of tutorial classes. In laboratory-based disciplines, the disparity between income and costs had been rising progressively.

The gap between income for research and for teaching Australian undergraduates and the costs was made up by income from international students. The fees charged to these students and their numbers were not regulated by government. The number of international students had been rising over the decade before I became vice-chancellor in 2003, and Australia-wide, about one quarter of university students were from overseas. The demographic had changed during this time, with the proportion of students from mainland China rising markedly with a gradual decrease in the proportion from South-East Asia. Large numbers of students were now coming from China, and to a lesser extent from India, to study in all faculties, but with the largest number in business and economics. Although the proportion of international students in information technology (IT) was still high, the absolute number had declined quite dramatically along with the number of Australian students enrolling in IT following the recent crash of the dot.com boom.

SCM, therefore, made it clear that if there was to be a growing research and research training effort at Monash University, there would have to be explicit cross-subsidisation of the expensive laboratory-based research areas in medicine, science and engineering by the faculties generating large incomes from international students and where research was less extensive and less expensive. The main source of this cross-subsidisation was the Faculty of Business and Economics. This, of course, led to considerable resentment and at times resistance by this faculty. Its staff were having to work harder and harder to educate more and more international students to cross-subsidise other faculties. This situation was being replicated across the country, although its extent was more visible at Monash, because of its SCM system, which made the cross-subsidy very transparent.

Overall, the budgeting process at Monash was more efficient and, I think, equitable than at the University of Melbourne at that time and after a lengthy process usually led to at least a grudging acceptance of outcomes and applause for the indomitable Reynold Dias, who managed the process. Gradual adjustments to the SCM model were made to provide the right incentives to faculties, but there were still arbitrary decisions to be made each year about the extent of the surpluses which each faculty was required to generate to contribute towards the costs of new capital expenditure.

Of course, each year when the budget situation appeared to be even more difficult than the year before, the spotlight fell on areas which were regarded as contributing to the problem. Notable amongst these were the campus in South Africa, the Gippsland campus and, for a number of years, the Faculty of Information Techology. Radical steps were taken to reduce staff numbers in the Faculty of Information Technology and to restructure its course offerings. Gradually, the numbers of students rose again and pressure came off that faculty, but South Africa and Gippsland remained major sources of controversy.

A feature of the approach that Alison Crook and the finance committee of council had taken was to borrow much more extensively than was usual in the Australian university context to fund new capital initiatives. In corporate terms, the borrowings were modest in relation to the financial position of the university. My new vice-president (finance), David Pitt, and I continued this process, but always kept within certain guidelines when doing so.

Borrowings did not exceed 25 per cent of annual revenue and there were always realisable reserves invested by Monash University or its foundation which would fully cover the borrowings, even allowing for a market downturn. The return on these investments more than covered the cost of borrowing, even allowing for the global financial crisis of 2008. Borrowings were never used to fund operating costs. The strategy worked because universities were regarded by the banks as excellent risks, so we were able to borrow at very fine margins. I was grateful to Alison Crook and David Pitt and to council for embracing this policy, as it freed up funding for major and needed capital development.

Another area which required attention from the administrative point of view was the corporate structure of Monash. During the turbulent Robinson days, it had been decided that the university was too large and inefficient to undertake some of its activities which required interaction with the private sector. Alison Crook and her colleagues had established incorporated controlled entities to run property and building developments (Monash Property Management, MPM), research commercialisation (MonCom), international student feeder education and English programs (Monash College) and a joint company with the student associations to run

CHAPTER 21

student services (Monyx). At the time, these separate company structures served a purpose and achieved a great deal. However, by the time I became vice-chancellor, whatever advantages there were in this separate structure were outweighed by the cumbersome governance, compliance and reporting requirements and the ambiguous role of the boards of the entities. On the one hand, they were meant to act in the interests of the entity they oversaw, whereas on the other hand, they were meant to be serving the interests of the controlling entity, Monash University.

The separate company structure meant that although the council of the university retained legal responsibility for the entities, its direct influence was buffered by the intervening board of the entity. At the management level, the separate corporate structures also created ambiguities in terms of responsibility and accountability. Divisions within the university, such as Facilities and Services, were often in apparent competition with corporate entities, such as Monash Property Management. The companies had also been formed on the assumption that divisions within the university could not assume the efficiency and nimbleness required to serve the university appropriately. I felt that the university had to be able to develop such abilities within its own structures. Moreover, the senior management of the corporate entities had been employed at top commercial rates, and the extra layer of management was costing the university a good deal. Following Alison Crook's retirement from Monash, the entities, apart from Monash College, were gradually dissolved and brought back into the university.

A central question facing all vice-chancellors is the senior management structure. At most universities in North America, the president (vice-chancellor) of the university has a senior deputy and has the deans reporting through that person, usually styled a provost. The provost is in charge of much or all of the internal management of the university, including teaching and research. The president's focus is then to a large extent external, building relationships with government, international partnerships and, most importantly, potential donors. The president may have vice-presidents (deputy vice-chancellors) reporting to him or her, or these too may report through the provost.

I considered such a structure, and I know that the senior deputy vice-chancellor Stephen Parker would have welcomed it. But given the timing and particularly taking account of the recent unrest at the university, I felt it was important that my focus should be, to a large extent, on matters internal to the university. I felt that the deans were central to getting the university united in its efforts to once more focus on excellence in education and research and in lifting the morale of the university. So I opted for a very flat structure, with the six deputy vice-chancellors and vice-presidents, the ten deans, the three pro vice-chancellors heading the Gippsland, Malaysian and South African campuses, the director of external relations and the director of the Monash University Museum of Art all reporting to me. I made it clear that the deans could and should deal directly with the appropriate deputy vice-chancellors for matters relating to education, research or international affairs, but that I would meet with them regularly and be responsible for their performance appraisals and overall line management.

Given all my other responsibilities relating to external relations, visiting and communicating with our widespread campuses, reporting to the council and general strategy and policy development, this made me extremely busy. It also gave me an excellent insight into the university and a knowledge of what was working and what was not. While I think this structure was right for me at that time, I do not pretend that such a flat structure is appropriate for such a large university into the future and I note that my successor as vice-chancellor, Ed Byrne, has recently appointed Edwina Cornish as the provost, with much of the responsibility for internal management of the university.

David Robinson had relied on the Vice-Chancellor's Group (VCG, essentially the deputy vice-chancellors) and the Committee of Deans as his major administrative committees. Given my conviction that the university needed high quality, committed and engaged senior administrative personnel in addition to the academic leaders, I created a larger group which we called the Senior Management Committee, comprising the VCG, deans and the heads of administrative divisions – about thirty in all), chaired by Stephen Parker, the senior deputy vice-chancellor. Although this inclusiveness worked to some extent, it was difficult to define its agenda separately from the Committee of Deans, and having a different chair created confusion. We later made the Committee of Deans an informal sounding-board, and I took over as chair of the Senior Management Committee, which became the major forum for the deans and the divisional heads.

Another issue to resolve was the role and status of the academic board. As instituted when Monash was founded, it was chaired by the vice-chancellor. In David Robinson's time, he passed this role to the deputy

CHAPTER 21

vice-chancellor (academic), Alan Lindsay. It was poorly attended and had neither the stature of a committee chaired by the vice-chancellor or the independence of a committee chaired by an elected president, a model I was familiar with at Melbourne and which pertained in most Australian universities. With the support of VCG and the academic board, I moved to the model of an elected president and Chris Browne from the Faculty of Medicine, Nursing and Health Sciences was elected as the initial president and did an excellent job.

Over time, particularly under the determined leadership of Jayne Godfrey, the academic board became an important 'house of review', ensuring that the academic staff of the university was supportive of changes initiated by senior management, and, through its committees working with the appropriate deputy vice-chancellors, initiating and implementing plans for education, research and international activities.

These steps reflected a move towards a greater degree of 'democratisation' of the process of management of the university. Although this was against the modern trend, I felt it was an important step towards restoring the confidence of the academic staff in the management and direction of the university, which had taken a battering in recent years.

By the time I left Monash, I felt that we had the best senior management team in any university in Australia and a committee structure that achieved an appropriate blend of efficiency and participation.

Work still to be completed included an improvement of the performance-appraisal system so that it became a system orientated to performance development and career support rather than to appraisal and greater flexibility in the definition of academic roles.

Although the academics' position description traditionally allocated about one third of the time to research, one third to teaching and one third to administrative and community engagement roles, it is quite clear that in order to achieve maximum contribution from the academic workforce, considerably more flexibility is required. Some staff are more suited to and capable of world class research and scholarship. Others may be passionate and innovative educators with less interest in research. These interests and aptitudes often change over an academic's career. The performance development framework must provide an environment for the supervisor to work with each individual to decide what proportion of his or her time should be devoted to teaching, research, administration and community engagement. Similarly, criteria for academic promotion should be flexible enough to reflect each individual's agreed profile.

I do not think that the extremes in a research university should extend to teaching only or research only academics. There might be teaching predominant (say 90 per cent teaching) and research predominant (say 90 per cent research) positions, but all should be committed to the shared objectives of the university in research and education and the nexus between the two. Similarly, flexibility between individuals and over professional lifetimes in administrative and community engagement activities should be retained.

Provided all activities are performed at a high level, they should be equally valued and rewarded. A good university excels at all these activities, and staff contributing at a high level to all these roles should be celebrated.

Another aspect of human resources related to the process of negotiating an enterprise agreement (or EBA) and the degree to which appointments would be made outside this agreement. Shortly after I started at Monash in September 2003, negotiations for the next EBA commenced. This was accompanied by stop-work meetings and staff pickets, although only a minority of staff participated. My intuitive approach was to say that it was in the university's interests to pay the people who worked there the highest amount that was compatible with sound financial management, and it was in the interests of the staff not to ask for salaries that would place the future of the university at risk. I was all for moving to our bottom line and saying this was the best and last offer. Our very experienced and wise head of human resources, Peter Marshall, soon to become vice-president of administration, provided wise counsel. The union had to be able to claim victories, or its standing would suffer. It could not let this happen so would fight tooth and nail to oppose the offer. On the other hand, if we offered less and were persuaded by the strong stance of the union to move our position towards that of the union, an honourable compromise could be reached and everyone would be happy. The other tactic was to let a deputy vice-chancellor and Peter, as the director of human resources, do the negotiation and for me to come in at the final stage with a more generous and final offer. Stephen Parker and Peter Marshall did a great job as the initial negotiators and encouraged me to come in as the 'white knight' at the final stage. A protracted process achieved the outcome that both the union and VCG would have settled for at the beginning. It took many hours of painstaking negotiation to reach this point, but honour was satisfied on both sides.

CHAPTER 21

This process was repeated when the next EBA was due in five years. My industrial relations knowledge had been upgraded.

An overarching principle I used throughout my time at Monash was that the essential role of senior management was to enable those at the coal face to deliver the highest quality education and the most innovative and contributory research that the university could hope to achieve. For this to occur, red tape had to be minimised, communication optimised and morale elevated so that the academic community could feel truly supported with an administration that shared their values and sought to allow their objectives to be achieved.

In every institution and organisational structure with which I have been associated, the biggest challenge has been communication. Whenever staff are asked to give feedback on institutional performance, the poorest performance is usually judged to be in communication. No matter how hard you try, this remains the major complaint. This does not mean that you should stop trying. Rather, you should try harder still and be philosophical about the fact that there will still be complaints.

I tried several techniques at Monash. The first was to ask the deans to ensure that they passed on information they learnt during the committee of deans, senior management committee and academic board to all the staff in their faculties. This tactic was to a large extent ineffective, because communication channels between the deans and their staff in big faculties were usually poorly developed, and in all faculties, the messages were often distorted. On many occasions, I was very surprised to hear back from academic or junior staff statements that I was reported to have made or opinions I was supposed to hold which were a distant highly distorted shadow of the original sentiment I had expressed. My tendency for informal and off-the-cuff comments, which were meant to be taken as humorous asides, were often reported back to me as strong statements of my opinion or policy. I should have learnt to be more careful, but that was not my nature. I needed a more direct way to speak to the university community.

I responded to all invitations to meet with and address individual campuses, faculties, schools or departments whenever it was possible to do so. These sessions were always valuable to me and I felt helped those I addressed to understand that I shared their commitment to research and education and understood or was keen to understand the constraints under which they operated. But even with the best will in the world, with 7000 staff and over 60,000 students, this direct communication approach reached only a small proportion of the staff and students. I was aware that global emails had to be handled very carefully. They could very easily sound like 'sermons from the mount' and make the vice-chancellor seem even more remote, out of touch and distant.

I decided that the most effective avenue I could use was the monthly *Monash Memo*, originally published in hard copy but then entirely online. I thought that the university's motto 'Ancora Imparo' (I am still learning) would be an appropriate title on two levels. In these monthly columns, I was able to communicate with those of the university community who were interested in matters relating to the latest higher education politics, in recent achievements of the university's staff or students, in research and education, and in my general philosophy about education and research and the role of universities such as Monash. I attempted to strike a balance between pomposity and triviality. In the last three years or so, these columns were broadcast, as well as appearing online, initially by Monash Radio and later by video. I found it difficult to avoid looking a bit robotic in the videos, reading from the autocue. I think I became a bit better at it over time, but by no means was I equipped for a career on TV.

Chapter 22

RESEARCH AND SCHOLARSHIP

One critical position requiring urgent renewal was that of the deputy vice-chancellor and vice-president (research). In its first twenty-five years or so, the university had established an excellent record in research and scholarship, particularly in areas such as engineering, chemistry, medicine, law and history. There was a perception, backed up by its recent performance in attracting nationally competitive grants from the Australian Research Council (ARC) and the National Health and Medical Research Council (NHMRC), that Monash had fallen behind the other Group of Eight universities in research. Perhaps its focus on the amalgamations that led to its huge expansion in the 1990s and its international ventures in Malaysia, South Africa and Italy had deflected its energy from research and scholarship to accommodating this rapid growth. There was certainly a strong feeling amongst some of the old hands at Monash that this was the case.

A defining element for me was the recruitment of Edwina Cornish as the deputy vice-chancellor and vice-president (research). She had been the deputy vice-chancellor (research) at the University of Adelaide and had in a short time earned a reputation for reinvigorating the research culture of that institution, which was also considered to be in the doldrums from the research point of view. Before that, she had worked for a number of years as the CEO of Florigene, a commercial company working on genetic manipulation of plants to produce new and exciting variants of traditional flower varieties. I felt that this commercial experience would stand us in good stead as we attempted not only to improve basic research performance, but also to work strategically in partnership with industry.

Edwina turned out to be inspirational in her role. She combined a unique blend of frankness, directness, toughness and charm. She was totally committed to research excellence and in a short time Monash was recognised as having transformed its research agenda. Moreover, Edwina worked strategically to develop or strengthen effective multidisciplinary groupings in areas of importance, such as sustainability, green chemistry, global movements, injury research and, most recently, regenerative medicine. Major research platforms to support outstanding research groups were acquired in protein crystallography, electron microscopy, advanced light microscopy, medical imaging, including a new medical beamline for the synchrotron, and a zebrafish core facility for regenerative medicine. Outstanding researchers were recruited. Edwina worked with the deans in a highly constructive but tough way. A new term, to be 'Cornished', was coined to describe an interaction between Edwina and a dean that centred around strong encouragement of the dean to improve the research performance of his or her faculty by encouraging more research grant applications, recruitment of research stars and improved mentoring and development of young researchers. Importantly, although Edwina's background was in the life sciences, the emphasis on improved performance of the university in research extended equally to scholarly work in the humanities and social sciences.

Edwina and I both felt that rather than defining in advance areas in which we should focus research effort, it was better to identify research stars and to support them with the equipment they needed and to recruit additional researchers in their area to make it a real research strength. Our objective was to reduce the red tape and to provide an enabling environment which would allow the best people to excel.

One of the most rewarding moments came when one of the outstanding young researchers at Monash was awarded the Science Minister's Prize for Research in the Life Sciences. James Whisstock stated, when he received his award, that he could do research at Monash that he would not be able to do anywhere else in the world. Given that he had received his PhD at Cambridge University and was very much a global citizen, this was a very significant comment. He was not referring solely to the infrastructure around him, although as he was a structural biologist, the protein crystallography facility and the synchrotron were invaluable. He was also referring to the freedom he had been given in his thirties to lead a research group and to be supported in his research by the resources of the university. His colleague, Jamie Rossjohn, originally from Cardiff

CHAPTER 22

University, who was also a protein crystallographer and had been similarly awarded with national prizes and a Federation Fellowship, shared his views. Both were sought by universities and research institutes around the world but preferred to stay at Monash.

The research performance of Monash University, which had been languishing, improved dramatically under Edwina's leadership. Significantly, this was across the different disciplines, with ARC funding as well as NHMRC funding increasing by large percentages in the years after Edwina was appointed.

Apart from the two outstanding researchers working independently in protein crystallography, there was great strength in other areas of basic medical research, especially microbiology and stem cell science, in some parts of pharmacy, in 'green' chemistry, in other parts of chemistry, in accident research, in chemical, materials and mechanical engineering, in some areas of law, particularly human rights law and mental health law, some areas of economics, particularly econometrics, and in history. Climate and environmental research was strong but scattered, and there was some interesting work in globalisation and global movements which was clearly relevant to Monash's aspiration to be a global university. Of course, there were many outstanding researchers in other areas, some working in groups and some in isolation.

The challenge for large universities such as Monash is to determine how much support to give to the strong areas of research to make them truly internationally competitive and how much to bolster the weaker areas. Despite the mantra that one university cannot be competitive in every area and therefore each university should focus on its areas of research strength, in a large and diverse university it is not appropriate to let important areas languish. For example, Edwina was of the view that an institution cannot be a world-class university without a strong physics department. Similar arguments can be made about some key areas in the humanities, mathematics and, of course, given the importance of school education to the future of the country, in education. Although one could strive to develop strong teaching departments in these areas without strong research, we were committed to the view that Monash should be a university where teaching was research-led and where the best teachers were also active researchers.

We therefore attempted to provide the most support we could to strong areas and to bolster those disciplines we felt were important but which were currently underperforming.

Another imperative was to assemble multidisciplinary teams to focus on some of the big issues of the time. Work had already begun on this with the Monash Institute for Global Movements, the Centre for Green Chemistry and the Monash University Accident Research Centre. New initiatives included the development of the Monash Sustainability Institute and the Australian Regenerative Medicine Institute and the Monash Institute for Pharmaceutical Sciences amongst others. The existing centres and institutes were strengthened. Some were very successful, others less so. The management of institutes and centres with personnel from different faculties, schools and departments requires considerable flexibility and goodwill. Essentially, there is a matrix structure, with a primary responsibility to the employing school or department and a 'dotted line' accountability to the head of the centre or institute. For those who were more comfortable with a single line of responsibility and accountability, this was a difficult structure to accommodate, but some form of matrix structure is inevitable in all large organisations with multiple lines of activity and geographic locations.

Another part of the vision that Edwina and I shared was that collaboration with other institutions was a more constructive and rewarding way to achieve results in research than trying to compete without deliberately working on collaborative relationships. This was a major rationale for many of the international initiatives already undertaken by Monash and further developed over the years to come. An immediate priority, however, was the relationship with two institutions in Melbourne, the University of Melbourne and CSIRO.

David Robinson and the vice-chancellor of the University of Melbourne, Alan Gilbert, had recognised the importance of Monash and the University of Melbourne working together and had jointly signed a memorandum of understanding known as the 'Melbourne-Monash protocol'. A few meetings between respective deans were undertaken and some joint activities resulted, but by 2003 there was little obvious impact of the protocol, apart from an annual golf match between senior management of the two universities.

It was clear that there was a significant feeling of envy towards the prestige occupied by Melbourne and its research record that at times almost seemed to amount to paranoia by some of the senior staff at

CHAPTER 22

Monash. Of course, there were many examples of active and successful collaborations between researchers in many fields, and there was frequent interchange of academic staff between the two institutions. Even so, I felt that the protocol needed to be reactivated, and when Glyn Davis took up his position as the vice-chancellor of the University of Melbourne, I called him. After having coffee together, we decided to have a research symposium to bring together researchers from the two universities around five themes covering different disciplines. This was held at the MCG and followed by a dinner.

Goodwill was expressed by all involved and a joint program in water management resulted. Other connections were made and collaborations continue to flourish, but understandably, there remains an ongoing atmosphere of competition between the two universities, perhaps most evident at Monash.

The relationship with CSIRO was one that Edwina and I felt was vital to the future of Monash. The largest campus of CSIRO was collocated with our Clayton campus and included the light metals flagship, clean coal technology, other areas of engineering and logistics. Over the years, there had been significant collaboration with researchers at Monash, but this had not been developed to the extent we felt it should.

As an initial step towards improving the dialogue, I phoned the CEO of CSIRO, Dr Geoff Garrett, and suggested we should have a dinner involving the senior researchers at both institutions. This was held and both Geoff and I expressed our view that we should work more closely together. As an initial and symbolic step, I suggested that the cyclone wire fence, which starkly demarcated the boundary between Monash and CSIRO, could be removed.

It took a number of years, but this eventually was achieved. More importantly, there has been a steady increase in the collaboration between Monash University and CSIRO. This culminated in a joint bid to the Education Investment Fund for a major contribution for a substantial new building costing about AUS$180 million on the Monash site adjoining CSIRO. This bid was successful and the building is now complete. Monash and CSIRO scientists will be working side by side on areas such as clean energy, materials, biomedical engineering, water and other areas of mutual strength. Research collaboration and PhD student supervision will be greatly enhanced, and the real potential of the two organisations to contribute significant research outcomes in these important areas will be enhanced.

The collocation of this major campus of CSIRO and the Clayton campus of Monash provided the opportunity for these organisations to form the hub of a technology and light manufacturing precinct. This had indeed evolved with this area of south-east Melbourne extending to Dandenong, being the home of light manufacturing and technology-based companies. The level of interaction between these companies and Monash University was variable. Some, such as the Wilson Transformer Company, had had a mutually rewarding association with Monash University since the 1960s. The Wilson Transformer Company has in many ways been a model Australian company, in that it has continuously evolved its technology in partnership with the engineering faculty at Monash and remained internationally competitive, including in a recent contract to install new transformers in the city of London. The technologists at Wilsons would come to the faculty at Monash and identify a problem they needed to address. Together, the technology would be developed to solve the problem. Of course, many Monash graduates worked at Wilsons and students were able to get work experience there.

This is a wonderful example of 'demand-driven' partnership between industry and a university. By and large, this is a more successful way to commercialise research than the occasional windfall that comes from commercialising the outcome of more basic research at a university. The 'supply-driven' process often manifested by the establishment of a 'spin-out' company to commercialise the discovery or by selling a licence to a company to do so, has been too great a focus for universities until recently. Monash University had a wholly owned company, MonCom, which had the role of managing Monash's research commercialising activities. As in the case of many other universities, this model was not successful. The separate company structure and a perceived or real pressure to be seen to be active and successful led to the development of a range of KPIs which encouraged certain lines of activity, which were not in the interests of the university or of the economic activity of the country. These included patents granted and 'spin-out' companies generated. Many of these patents amounted to nothing, and many of the spin-out companies foundered.

Edwina and I felt that we should bring the commercial activity back into the main university structure and focus on partnerships with industry that

CHAPTER 22

were mutually beneficial. This did not mean that, where it was appropriate to do so, the basic discoveries with commercial potential should not be patented or that every effort should not be made to realise the commercial return from such discoveries. By and large, however, universities were not well set up to start a company, and a licensing or royalty arrangement usually made more sense.

Having said that, Monash University was the beneficiary of what was perhaps the most successful commercialisation activity by any university in Australia. Under the direction of the foundation professor of obstetrics and gynaecology, Carl Wood, and with research driven by Alan Trounson, working with John Leeton, Gab Kovacs and Alex Lopata and collaborating with Ian Johnston at the Royal Women's Hospital, Monash University was a world leader in the introduction of in vitro fertilisation to humans. Research at Monash led to the use of hormones to greatly increase the success rate of IVF, use of frozen embryos and a number of other innovations. The doctors and scientists involved had the foresight to establish a company, later known as Monash IVF, to deliver IVF services and to conduct further research into infertility treatment. For many years, the company was not profitable, but from the beginning of the decade, it was delivering a dividend of several million dollars per year to Monash, which owned 53 per cent of the company.

Stephen Parker initially, and then David Pitt, the vice-president of finance, chaired the board of Monash IVF. Neither David nor I felt it appropriate for a university to be in effective and ongoing control of a company delivering clinical services. There was risk involved and the relationship with the doctors delivering the services was often fractious.

After a protracted period of negotiations, the board decided to sell Monash IVF to a private equity company. Monash University's share of the proceeds was just over AUS$100 million, a considerable windfall. David Pitt was smart enough to see that the global financial situation was at best uncertain and invested the proceeds as cash just before the global financial crisis of 2008 greatly reduced the value of other forms of investment.

Edwina and I were keen to develop a more constructive relationship with potential industry partners. This led to the appointment of a pro vice-chancellor (industry engagement and commercialisation). Professor Rod Hill, a senior scientist and administrator at CSIRO, was appointed to this position and has increased the ability of Monash to engage with industry and for private companies to engage with Monash. Much remains to be achieved in terms of optimising what should be a mutually rewarding partnership between Monash and industry, but progress is being made.

The vision of a major hub of innovation and industry based around Monash University and CSIRO at Clayton, the adjoining Australian Synchrotron and the Melbourne Centre for Nanofabrication remains to be fully realised, but with visionary government and private investment, this precinct has the potential to be an economic driver of great significance to Victoria and Australia. The future of manufacturing in Australia lies in innovation founded on research with industry, working in partnership with universities and CSIRO to produce niche products to export to a global market.

Chapter 23

EDUCATION

One of the unfortunate accompaniments of the emphasis that has been placed in recent years on world rankings of universities is the relative neglect of the quality of the education delivered by the university. Although analysis of publications, including citation rates, and international awards such as Nobel Prizes to graduates and staff allows objective (although not necessarily valid) measures of relative performance of universities in research and scholarship, no such measures exist for the quality of education in universities. Attempts to establish such measures in Australia to allow allocation of funds from the government's Learning and Teaching Performance Fund for a few years in the first decade of the twenty-first century used surrogates. These included the retrospective evaluation by new graduates of their educational experience at the university in the course-evaluation questionnaire, progression rates and success of graduates in obtaining employment. It is a moot point whether these criteria gave much information about the quality of the educational experience of students, and once they were used to determine funding, they were potentially subject to 'gaming' by the universities.

The lack of objective measures for the quality of education and the perceived emphasis given to research performance in determining promotion led to a perception by the staff that education and their performance as educators were not valued by universities.

From the beginning of my time as vice-chancellor, I emphasised that it was equally important for the university to excel in education as in research and scholarship. Even if the quality of the educational experience did not feed into the international ranking and reputation of the university, all staff had a duty of care to the 60,000 students who had entrusted their tertiary education and research training to us. We had an absolute obligation to ensure that the quality of the educational experience was as high as it possibly could be.

I liked to describe education and research as the twin peaks of our endeavours as a university. We could not claim to be a great university unless we were excellent at both. They are interdependent with a key component of the educational process being the instillation of the curiosity and ability to discover information that is the basis of research. The oft-referred-to nexus between teaching and research had to be real and express itself as research-led teaching. Given that information was now ubiquitous and readily accessible, university education had to be about more than the transmission and organisation of this information into usable knowledge. It must also develop the important higher order generic skills of creativity, critical analysis, problem-solving, teamwork and communication. These same skills underpin research.

During my time at Monash, we all worked hard to give education the priority it deserved. I spoke of it often; we awarded vice-chancellor's prizes each year for the best teachers at different levels and encouraged active participation in the Australian Learning and Teaching Council Awards. Under the leadership of Graham Webb, the pro vice-chancellor (quality), we introduced routine and mandatory student questionnaires for each unit of study and at the faculty operational performance reviews we followed up the actions taken to address units where the educational experience of students was ranked as poor by the students.

Of course, the word-of-mouth (or social media) evaluation of the educational experience of students was important in retaining and increasing the ability of universities to attract students, both Australian and international. It therefore flowed into the overall financial health and reputation of the university, so the emphasis on the quality of education was not entirely altruistic.

Education at all levels is undergoing dramatic changes. The advances in information and communications technology have and will continue to have dramatic effects on not only the education process but also on the very purpose of that education. Although good educationalists would have argued for centuries that education is about opening minds, stimulating curiosity and increasing the ability of individuals to continue to learn over their lifetimes, too often the process has been the transfer of information to increase the knowledge bank of the student to be reproduced uncritically in the examination process. Rote learning for the examinations was a test of memory and application but hardly a preparation for a productive and enjoyable life marked by creativity, curiosity and lifelong learning.

Lectures can be recorded and accessed online and laboratory classes can be simulated in real time using digital tablets. There is an almost limitless supply of educational materials, images and videos available online and some prestigious universities are providing open access to whole courses on the internet. Students communicate widely with large groups not only in their own classes but with other young people around the world.

Monash had a particular need to utilise new technologies, given its multicampus structure and the relatively high proportion of its students at Gippsland who were not located close to the Churchill campus and who needed to undertake courses largely accessed off-site. There had already been a substantial distance education program, but much had been undertaken in written format, so transforming to digital technology was a big task. Limited bandwidth also restricted the ability to use the new technologies to reach into rural locations, and the speed of transmission to international sites such as South Africa, Malaysia and Italy impeded our efforts to have campuses optimally linked by digital technology. However, substantial progress has been made and is continuing to be made.

During my time at Monash, the University of Melbourne introduced what became known as the 'Melbourne model'. Essentially, the number of undergraduate degrees was reduced to six broadly based degrees (arts, biomedicine, commerce, environments, music and science). Professional degrees such as law, medicine, dentistry, physiotherapy, engineering, architecture, and so on, were then undertaken at the graduate level. Although having the theoretical advantage of allowing students more time to choose and the opportunity to undertake broad tertiary education before entering a professional course, it also prolonged the total duration required to undertake a professional degree and delayed the selection for competitive courses. This prevented definition of a clear career direction until much later. The professional requirements of a number of the professional accrediting bodies obliged students to undertake one or another of the undergraduate degrees, such as biomedicine for medicine, environments for architecture and science for engineering. This tended to militate against the idea of a broad education before choosing a professional degree. At postgraduate level, it is possible for universities to set fees in an unregulated (albeit competitive) environment.

Although not suggesting that this motivated the University of Melbourne, a perverse incentive to move professional degrees to postgraduate level will continue as long as undergraduate fees are regulated by government.

Although having potential financial advantages for the university, my colleagues and I did not support introducing the Melbourne model at Monash. We felt that lengthening the time required to undertake a basic professional degree was not in the community's interests and not what most students wanted. For example, if you wanted to do a medical degree and were offered a place at Monash which would take five years, why would you choose a place in biomedicine at Melbourne, compete for entry to medicine after three years, be exposed to the possibility of full fees and another four years of study to become a doctor. Similar arguments applied to the other professional disciplines.

There were some very positive aspects of the undergraduate program at Monash. Dual degrees were common with a lot of flexibility about the disciplines which were combined. Medicine offered the option of a year of research for a second degree (BMedSci), with the total duration still being one year less than the time taken to get a basic medical qualification under the Melbourne model. There was considerable flexibility with respect to students transferring between different courses and carrying credit across.

So we were very happy to continue to work with our direct undergraduate entry to professional as well as general courses while providing the option of graduate entry as well. This decision has clearly been vindicated in the students' minds with Monash University being not only the most popular first-choice university for Victorian school-leavers, but also the most popular for the highest achieving school-leavers (i.e. Australian Tertiary Admission Rank in the top 5 per cent).

This did not mean that change in the way the programs were delivered was not required. There was also a requirement to greatly reduce the number of units and courses offered which, as in other universities, had tended to proliferate without check. Academics have an understandable inclination to want to teach courses in their area of scholarly interest, so new, specialised units (subjects) tend to be developed, driven by the passion of an individual lecturer. If that academic then leaves, the unit remains as an offering for students to choose. The number of students dwindles, the academic staff no longer has any champion for the area and the quality of the educational experience declines. About half the total units offered at Monash fell into this category with a very small number of students taking them. So the approaches were to sharpen the unit and course offerings by removing the poor quality, low demand units and courses, preserving the popular and high-quality courses and increasing the demand for the high quality, relevant units and courses which were poorly subscribed. Of course, each removal of a unit or course was fiercely opposed by a small number of devotees or those ideologically opposed to any perceived reduction in choice, particularly in the humanities.

Adam Shoemaker, who was appointed to the role of deputy vice-chancellor (education) when Stephen Parker left to become vice-chancellor of the University of Canberra, wanted the undergraduate offerings at Monash to be innovative and highly attractive to the students. He saw the opportunity to take advantage of our global campuses and relationships and also our reputation and emphasis on social justice. The latter was exemplified by the formation by Monash students led by the remarkable Hugh Evans of the Oaktree Foundation, an international community development program managed by young people (aged under twenty-five), which has become a global organisation with many thousands of members.

Adam packaged the particular educational programs at Monash as the Monash Passport. This carried the implication both of being international and of enabling entry to any field of endeavour.

The components of the Monash Passport are:

- action through volunteer programs, community engagement and work-integrated learning
- enhancement through depth subjects and other programs preparing the student to be a critical and creative thinker who can produce innovative solutions to multifaceted problems or to be a future leader
- exploration through international experiences and perspectives by study abroad or collaboration between Monash's Australian and international campuses
- investigation through encouragement of the student to develop research skills and discover new knowledge through research challenge units or vacation research projects.

Of course, there had already been evolution of teaching methodologies and course content to develop the opportunities inherent in the Monash Passport concept, but the packaging and badging of the components made it clear to prospective students and the general community that Monash was aware of the challenges and opportunities provided by the educational transition associated with the advances in educational technology and the demands of the rapidly evolving and globalised work environment of the twenty-first century. The components of the passport emphasised the need for self-directed learning, innovation and creativity, teamwork and communication, commitment to others and an international perspective.

The strong demand by domestic and international students for Monash University demonstrates that the university has been very successful providing educational opportunities that appeal to students. The strong demand for Monash graduates in the workplace shows that the university is equipping its graduates with skills and abilities which employers appreciate, both in Australia and internationally.

Chapter 24

THE VICTORIAN CAMPUSES OF MONASH UNIVERSITY

Soon after I was appointed as vice-chancellor at Monash, it became clear to me that issues around the multicampus structure of Monash in Victoria were still unresolved more than ten years after the amalgamation of the Chisholm Institute (Caulfield and Frankston) to form the Caulfield and Peninsula campuses of Monash University and the amalgamation with the Gippsland College of Advanced Education to form the Gippsland campus. It was eight years since the university was granted the land in Berwick to develop the Berwick campus.

The amalgamations had occurred as a result of the so-called Dawkins Reforms of the higher education system to move to a unitary system. Many of the academic staff who had worked so hard to establish the reputation of Monash University as a top international research university were dismayed that this research standing would be undermined by the amalgamation with the Chisholm campuses and Gippsland, which, although worthy educational institutions, did not have a research culture. Most of their teaching staff had no research pretensions and many did not have a PhD. Moreover, there were major ideological differences between the David Syme Business School at Caulfield and the Faculty of Economics and Commerce at Clayton. It was also felt that trying to establish a new campus at Berwick, just over twenty minutes on the Monash Freeway from the Clayton campus, was an expensive and distracting exercise and that the entry standards of Monash would have to be compromised if students were to be attracted to the campus.

My view was that the multicampus structure was here to stay and that it would not be politically acceptable or wise to challenge it. Moreover, if we were strategic, we could make this an advantage for Monash in an environment where governments were endeavouring to develop regional centres and to widen the opportunity for participation in higher education for people from the lowest socio-economic quartile who were currently substantially under-represented at university. We could not have five Claytons, but if we were clever, each campus could be developed in a way that it had particular strengths. We would expect Clayton, Caulfield and, in its specialist field, Parkville to undertake internationally relevant research, whereas Gippsland, Peninsula and Berwick would concentrate on niche areas of research, especially those relevant to the local community or specialist areas of strength. This research, although of lesser scope, should also be of excellent quality and provide opportunities for PhD training of high calibre.

Clayton, with its hosting of the Australian Synchrotron, its collocation with CSIRO and its central location in a vibrant area of light manufacturing and biomedical technology, would continue to evolve as a major site of engineering, scientific and biomedical research with continuing activity in its traditional areas of research and scholarship in the humanities and social sciences. It would remain the centre of university administration and, with its wonderful facilities, be the main centre for the performing arts, sports and ceremonial occasions.

The strength of the Clayton campus in the areas of engineering, science and biomedicine was reinforced not only by the commissioning of the synchrotron but also by the completion of a new medical science building with the help of the state and the commonwealth funding. There were plans for a major new building for engineering and science which would be shared with CSIRO staff building the relationship. A number of state of the art research platforms, including an electron microscopy facility, a robotic protein crystallography facility, a zebra fish core facility and an advanced light microscopy centre were developed. The support of the Bracks-Brumby state government is particularly acknowledged, together with funds from the Higher Education Endowment Fund.

The role of the Clayton campus as the headquarters of the science and technology disciplines at Monash has been enhanced by the state's first specialist science high school being built on the campus. Opened in 2009, it is a showpiece for science education and provides opportunities for bright students in the state system to experience the highest quality science education which is available. They also gain a taste of university life and the staff of the university engage with the school to inspire the students about science and about learning. It has been a great initiative.

CHAPTER 24

Although the Caulfield campus is compact, it is the primary site for about 13,000 students. It is the headquarters for the Faculty of Business and Economics and for the Faculty of Art and Design. The Faculty of Information Technology also has a substantial presence on that campus. Gradually, increasing components of the Faculty of Arts have also been relocated there, including the highly visible Centre for Jewish Civilisation. There is a relatively high percentage of international students. Given its proximity to the Caulfield railway station and the Dandenong Road trams, it is very accessible by public transport. A shuttle bus connects it with the Clayton campus. It is very popular with students and has an active and vibrant social life. Unlike the Clayton campus, student politics tend to be dominated by the conservatives, and this has led, from time to time to intense conflicts between the student unions and associations on the two campuses.

Given its previous life, initially as Caulfield Technical School and Caulfield Technical College and then Chisholm Institute, the more traditional academics tended to regard the Caulfield staff and the campus as of lesser status. In particular, there was a history of dispute and lack of mutual regard or respect between the staff of the Faculty of Business and Economics on the Caulfield campus and the Clayton campus. Even thirteen years after the merger, this had not totally subsided, although the situation was gradually improving and continued to do so during my time at Monash.

Two events relating to the Faculty of Art and Design were important in elevating the status of this campus so that it started to be viewed as an equal partner to the Clayton campus, or the 'original' Monash.

The first was the establishment of the School of Architecture by the Faculty of Art and Design. This was the first new school of architecture to be established in Australia for many years and was warmly welcomed and strongly supported by the profession. Originally, I had planned that it might be located on the Berwick campus, providing a strong and prestigious focus for that campus. However, consultation suggested that a location at Caulfield, along with other elements of the faculty, including those related to design, would make it much more likely to succeed and to appeal to the best students. The school took its first students in 2008 and has indeed been highly successful and popular under the guidance of its foundation professor, Shane Murray, and the then dean of the faculty, John Redmond.

The second initiative was to create a new gallery to house the Monash University Museum of Art and to make Caulfield the centre for visual arts, just as Clayton, with its wonderful facilities, was clearly the centre for performing arts.

The Monash University Museum of Art had a proud history. The early professors recognised the importance that a fine collection of art had for the cultural, educational and scholarly life of a university and for each new campus building a small amount of the capital expenditure was set aside for the purchase of works of art so that the new buildings could be appropriately embellished. Together with generous philanthropy and with the inspirational leadership of an early professor of fine arts, the redoubtable Patrick McCaughey, an impressive collection had been established representing the best of modern Australian art. A new building for the museum had been built in the late 1980s. Unfortunately, it was not adequate to provide an ongoing display of some of Monash's more significant works and also to provide a program of exhibitions to engage the community and to bring them to Monash.

There had been a somewhat fraught recent history of MUMA. Its director for many years before I came to Monash had been Jenepher Duncan, a highly respected figure amongst the arts community of Melbourne. There had been a feeling that MUMA had been catering too much to the elite end of the arts community and not engaging enough with the general community. Whatever the rights and wrongs of the situation, Ms Duncan had left and there was a lot of sympathy for her amongst her colleagues and the arts cognoscenti. Fortunately, her successor, Max Delaney, did a wonderful job in rebuilding the relations with the arts community and in running a highly successful exhibition program which succeeded in engaging with the general community. He and John Redmond – the dean of the Faculty of Art and Design, who chaired the MUMA advisory committee – both advocated for a new gallery constructed from refurbished space to provide a more spacious new home for MUMA on the Caulfield campus. Space was potentially available adjacent to the art and design building at Caulfield underneath the new architecture school. This space had become available with the consolidation of engineering to the Clayton campus.

Approximately AUS$7 million was required. This was raised by a combination of philanthropy and capital expenditure by Monash. The new gallery provides an excellent venue for displaying some of the permanent collection and for exhibitions and brings many members of the community including school groups to the Caulfield campus.

CHAPTER 24

The university council recognised Jenepher Duncan's outstanding contribution to the university with the award of an honorary degree.

The completion of a new building at Caulfield a little after I commenced allowed more of the arts faculty to relocate to the campus and for the Faculty of Business and Economics to be expanded and upgraded. Together with the commencement of architecture and the relocation of MUMA, it did much to make the Caulfield campus an equal partner with the larger but less accessible Clayton campus. However, the western or city end of the campus was still unimpressive and largely occupied by a variety of leased premises which together formed a shopping plaza. The largest part of this was a Coles supermarket, which was on an extended lease.

David Pitt, the vice-president (finance), Peter Marshall, the vice-president (administration) and I felt that we could achieve a number of objectives if we were to relocate the law school to that site and also provide more student accommodation. The law school was still located in its original building from the 1960s. As the home of the illustrious David Derham School of Law, the building was viewed with affection, but it was becoming overcrowded and not sufficiently up to date with the digitally connected world of the twenty-first century. We felt that providing a new building for the law school on the Caulfield campus would address these problems and make the law school more accessible from and connected with the city. Moreover, the law school building could be refurbished and made into an attractive new home for the education faculty.

A detailed proposal was developed with Equiset, by then under the leadership of Lorenz Grollo. The land would be transferred to Equiset, and a new law school building would be constructed along with substantial student accommodation and student facilities. Plans were drawn up, and after debate within the law school, the relocation was supported by the faculty.

Unfortunately, the global financial crisis then unfolded and funding was not available to make the project viable at that time. In a last-minute attempt to save the project, Lorenz flew me with him in the Grollo private plane to Canberra to speak with a number of ministers. Although they were supportive of the project and spoke vaguely of the need for it to be supported, there was no definite guarantee. After discussions with David Pitt, we decided to withdraw from the project as the deadline for achieving closure had passed.

The idea of relocation of the law school in a new building at Caulfield remains, but it will have to await more propitious times to bring it to fruition.

The Caulfield campus is now a highly regarded part of the Monash family and will grow further in importance over time.

The Gippsland campus was regarded as a particular challenge. Quite apart from its lack of a research culture, it was struggling to attract students and the introduction of activity-based costing had shown that it was losing about six million dollars per year. There was much nervousness at Gippsland about what the Monash administration might be planning for the campus and this nervousness had recently been exacerbated by the decision of the engineering faculty to withdraw from the campus and therefore not offer its bachelor of engineering degree. Instead, an engineering degree unique to the Gippsland campus was to be administered through a new school of applied science and engineering. The new degree to be titled bachelor of civil and environmental engineering would have a more general focus than the BEng that it replaced but represented a reversion to the model after merger where Gippsland degrees were identifiably different from those offered at Clayton.

The campus was very unhappy about this and feared that it may represent the beginning of a progressive decline of the campus. There was also industrial unrest resulting from some staffing consequences of the change and unrest amongst the students who had commenced the previous course and who had been told they must either relocate to Clayton or take the remainder of their course by distance education from the University of Southern Queensland.

I first visited the campus early in my days as vice-chancellor. It was clear to me that there were many committed staff and that the head of the campus, Pro Vice-Chancellor Brian McKenzie, had worked hard to build relations with the local community and industry. Its strategic location in the Latrobe Valley, in the heart of the power industry, meant that it would provide opportunities for partnerships and applied research. I also recognised from my experience at the University of Melbourne that it would be politically crazy to do anything but work to make the campus successful. It was the only significant regional university campus in eastern Victoria and given the government's enthusiasm to widen educational opportunity, any withdrawal of services would not be in the community's interest and would be politically unwise for the university. Having firmly come to this decision, I was asked to address a lunchtime gathering of senior community leaders and academics from the campus.

CHAPTER 24

To me, it was so obvious that it was in the university's interest to resolve the problems and to make the campus successful that I felt it safe to start with the obviously nonsensical statement that we planned to close the campus. That was received with a stunned silence. I quickly explained that I was joking and of course the campus was of such obvious benefit to Monash and to the local community that I was totally committed to it. Moreover, we would work with the staff and students to ensure that the campus became still more effective, further developing its research agenda to provide opportunities for high-quality PhD training and for research in fields relevant to the local community and industry.

We worked through the issue of the engineering students and committed to a program where they could be 'taught out' at the campus to allow them to complete the degree they had commenced. Industrial issues were negotiated through to a peaceful resolution and gradually the relationship between the campus and Clayton improved.

There was, however, a structural problem in administration, which meant that it would be very difficult for the campus to be sustainable over time. In the matrix model of administration, the faculties were responsible for the academic programs at Gippsland. The academic staff had primary affiliation with their faculties rather than with the campus. The pro vice-chancellor had no real levers to alter academic programs or to take new initiatives and had a limited dotted-line relationship with the academic staff. Although he was the figurehead for the campus, the ability of the pro vice-chancellor to respond to local needs in education and research depended on his ability to persuade the deans to support a particular initiative.

From the point of view of the deans, the relatively small scale of the operation at Gippsland compared with Clayton and Caulfield meant that in many cases it did not make financial sense for them to continue to support academic programs at Gippsland. Moreover, it was more difficult to attract and retain high-calibre staff, and the lesser competition for places meant that the entry standard for students was lower. Thus, although there may have been political and altruistic reasons for supporting the campus, it did not make a lot of sense from the point of view of deans responsible for the educational, research and financial performance of their faculties.

After much discussion, we decided that it would be best to alter the matrix structure to give the campus responsibility for its budget and the line-management responsibility for the academic staff and the delivery of the education and research programs. Thus the solid line of responsibility in the matrix structure would now be from the academic staff to the head of school at Gippsland and then to the pro vice-chancellor. A 'dotted line' accountability to the faculty through the head of school or department at Clayton or Caulfield and the dean of the faculty would signify the importance of retaining the quality control and involvement in the educational programs of the faculty.

This was generally welcomed at Gippsland. A number of the deans viewed it with dismay but eventually accepted it. The pro vice-chancellor, Brian McKenzie, worked hard to communicate and collaborate with the deans and when ill-health forced his retirement, the new pro vice-chancellor, Helen Bartlett, ensured that relationships with the faculties were developed as collaboratively as possible.

It was important that alternative entry pathways were developed to allow Monash Gippsland to provide tertiary education to local students who had had less educational opportunity to satisfy the traditional entry requirements for Monash. Partnerships were developed with the Gippsland College of TAFE and with the Kurnai Secondary College to form the Gippsland Educational Precinct. Pathways between TAFE courses and tertiary courses at Monash were developed and encouraged. A diploma of tertiary studies was offered by Monash as a foundation year with successful completion at a certain level, allowing entrance with credits to Monash. An associate degree structure was also developed with successful completion, allowing transition to completion of a full degree.

With a lot of hard work by the staff and by Helen Bartlett in particular, the budget position improved from a deficit of AUS$6 million per annum when the campus first became responsible for its own budget to a break-even budget by 2009.

A key development for the campus was the commencement of the new branch of the Monash medical school, headquartered at Monash University Gippsland. By the early 2000s, it had become apparent that the prevailing political and economic opinion that there were too many medical graduates was incorrect and that the opposite was true. More medical graduates were urgently needed. Existing medical schools were asked to take more students and new medical schools were created at a number of eager universities which believed that a medical school was essential if the university was

CHAPTER 24

to achieve appropriate prestige and recognition. In Victoria, Deakin University was awarded a medical school and Monash was successful in its bid to establish a graduate-entry medical school headquartered at its Gippsland campus.

Interestingly, we learnt a little about the political process in the lead up to being granted the medical school at Gippsland. The local member for the region was Peter McGauran, a cabinet minister. He was strongly supportive of the campus and we felt, with a friend in the cabinet, that as long as we gave him the appropriate strong arguments for the school, it should be straightforward. I went to visit him with Ed Byrne, the dean of the Faculty of Medicine, Nursing and Health Sciences and explained both the need for the school and the benefits for the campus as a whole. He said he was strongly in its favour, but said that we needed to engage a lobbyist so that his fellow cabinet ministers would be persuaded. He said that Sally Walker, the vice-chancellor of Deakin, had been marching the corridors of Parliament House with a lobbyist, and we needed to do the same.

One would have thought that a paid lobbyist would be less effective than a cabinet minister in making the case! We did what he advised and employed a lobbyist with links to the Liberal Party, and we were awarded the medical school at Gippsland.

The medical school took its first students in 2008, and they graduated at the end of 2011. The program has been highly successful.

Importantly, the medical school at Gippsland, together with the greater autonomy granted to it in controlling its budget and in academic management, signified the importance placed on the campus by the council and administrative leadership of Monash. It has gradually increased its research profile and has over 100 PhD students. It is not and will not be a replica of Clayton. But it is fulfilling an important regional role as a high-quality university campus, providing educational opportunity, not otherwise easily obtainable by local students, and applied research relevant to the region.

Debate continued about its role. Recently, the campus has been amalgamated with Ballarat University to form Federation University. The medical school remains part of Monash.

Each of the other Australian campuses presents its own particular challenges and opportunities.

The Peninsula campus had started life as a teachers' college at Frankston, becoming known in 1973 as the State College at Frankston. It had become the Frankston campus of the newly formed Chisholm Institute of Technology in 1982. The Caulfield and Frankston campuses of the Chisholm Institute formally amalgamated with Monash University on 1 July 1990.

Given its history, teacher education was initially its mainstay with a particular emphasis on early childhood and primary school education. There were also courses in accounting and business and economics. It was strategically located on a beautiful site at the gateway of the Mornington Peninsula with its growing population and active tourism industry.

At the first Monash senior management planning meeting I attended before taking up my appointment, the dean of the Faculty of Medicine, Nursing and Health Sciences, Nick Saunders, had suggested that the standing of the campus and its general attractiveness to students could be enhanced by locating two new health science courses there – physiotherapy and occupational therapy. There was a shortage of health care professionals in these disciplines, and courses in these areas were not offered anywhere in the south or eastern parts of Melbourne. Following Professor Saunders retirement, Ed Byrne became the new dean. He and I, together with VCG, decided to proceed with these initiatives. Dynamic young academics were appointed to head them and they have been highly successful. They have achieved their aim to increase the popularity and status of the campus. Nevertheless, the centripetal pull of the larger campuses remained a factor with the bachelor of health sciences relocating to Clayton. Adjustments also had to be made to the offerings in business and economics and IT due to difficulty in attracting sufficient students to make some of the courses viable on this campus.

The history of the Berwick campus was quite different. It had started life as the Casey airfield, initially privately owned by Lord Richard Casey, who had been governor-general of Australia from 1965 to 1969. It was taken over by commercial interests in 1968 and, with a lot of local advocacy, made available to Monash University in 1994 with the first buildings completed and students commencing in 1996.

The campus occupied a large area of fifty-six hectares, strategically located on the extension of the Monash Freeway and on the corridor linking Monash Clayton with Monash Gippsland. Berwick was the centre of one of the youngest and fastest growing population areas in Australia. It had an over-representation of people from the lower socio-economic groups and was poorly served with tertiary institutions. The percentage of school-leavers accessing higher education was well below the state and national

CHAPTER 24

average. A TAFE campus was located nearby, and the new Casey hospital had recently been completed across the road. It was well served by public transport.

It is a financial challenge to fund the capital development required for a new university campus. Alison Crook, the deputy vice-chancellor (resources) when I commenced, had been in dialogue with a commercial property developer to plan the joint academic, corporate and residential development of the campus. It was an innovative proposal which would have greatly accelerated the development of academic facilities, student accommodation and a variety of retail developments supplying the students' needs. There would be some commercial developments as well, with preference given to those which would work with the university.

There was nervousness amongst the Monash community about this proposal as some saw it as a threat to the academic integrity of the university. The local Berwick-Casey community were also anxious that it would essentially become a real estate development, and the prime purpose of providing opportunities for university access to local young people would become secondary. This concern was shared by Bob Charles, who as the local federal MP had been a major advocate of the proposal to make the airfield into a university campus. The state minister for education, Lynne Kosky, was also less than enthusiastic about the proposal.

We decided in the end not to proceed and instead to develop an alternative strategy. Central to this was the idea of an education precinct taking advantage of the adjacent TAFE campus and negotiating with the state government about the location of a planned new selective-entry high school for the south-eastern suburbs. Following the highly successful models of Melbourne High School and MacRobertson's High School, which granted entry by competition to high achieving boys and girls in the public system, it was planned that two new selective-entry high schools should be created to service the rapidly growing communities to the west (Wyndham) and south-east of Melbourne. It was decided, after discussion, that the Berwick campus of Monash would be the site of the school to the south east and that it would be called the Nossal High School after the highly esteemed and long-time director of the Walter and Eliza Hall Institute of Medical Research, Sir Gustav Nossal.

By making the campus the focus for some of the brightest high school students, we hoped that this would increase awareness of the opportunities for tertiary entrance, particularly to Monash University, either at the new facilities at Berwick or the more established campuses at Clayton, Caulfield or elsewhere.

The Nossal High School is now well and truly functioning and the campus is buzzing. Leon Piterman has taken over from Philip Steele as the pro vice-chancellor and is building on early work by many people to make the campus a vibrant member of the Monash family. The education faculty has taken advantage of the high school to establish activities on the campus and a number of other new initiatives, including health and ageing, have added to the earlier emphasis on small business, tourism and IT.

The Parkville campus is the home of the Faculty of Pharmacy and Pharmaceutical Sciences, previously known as the Pharmacy College. At the time of the Dawkins 'reforms' in the late 1980s, it was expected that the Pharmacy College would amalgamate with the University of Melbourne. But negotiations broke down. A key factor was the wish for the Pharmacy College to be a separate faculty, whereas the vice-chancellor, David Penington, and the dean of medicine, Graeme Ryan, said that it should be part of an expanded Faculty of Medicine, Dentistry and Health Sciences. Monash's vice-chancellor, Mal Logan, agreed to it becoming a separate faculty and the unlikely outcome of the college becoming part of Monash University eventuated.

From my point of view, having the Faculty of Pharmacy and Pharmaceutical Sciences located in Parkville was a great strategic advantage as it gave Monash University a home within the much-vaunted 'Parkville Strip', the home of several of Australia's leading medical research institutes, hospitals, and the University of Melbourne. It could only help the collaboration between Monash and the institutions of the Parkville strip. Indeed, when I was the dean of the Faculty of Medicine, Dentistry and Health Sciences at the University of Melbourne and we were establishing the Bio 21 Cluster, I encouraged the members to invite the Pharmacy College to join to maximise the collaboration.

The development of a new building for the faculty and the refurbishment of one of the major existing buildings provided opportunities for the faculty to lift its performance in research and education. A challenge was provided by the geographic separation of the Pharmacy College from the Clayton campus, particularly from biomedical science, including pharmacology, research and teaching.

CHAPTER 24

The long-standing dean of the faculty, Colin Chapman, had overseen the expansion of the teaching program of the faculty to include multidisciplinary programs in formulation science and pharmaceutical sciences, in addition to the traditional professional training degree in pharmacy. A pre-practice year had also been introduced. Research needed a boost, and the recruitment of Bill Charman and his team achieved this.

Under the dynamic leadership of Bill Charman, who succeeded Colin Chapman as dean in 2007, the faculty has gone from strength to strength. It has rapidly become the top-ranked pharmacy school in the country and the sixth-ranked school in the world in the QS ranking system. The highly successful Centre for Drug Candidate Optimisation, which received large amounts of funding both from the Victorian government and from the industry, has played an important role in the success of the faculty. The new building provided the opportunity for a multidisciplinary research centre known as the Monash Institute for Pharmaceutical Sciences. Two key researchers from the department of Pharmacology at Clayton relocated there and aided collaboration with biomedical sciences at Clayton.

The faculty now attracts large amounts of external funding from the pharmaceutical industry, the Bill and Melinda Gates Foundation, the Wellcome Trust, the Medicines for Malaria Venture of the WHO and traditional competitive funding sources such as NHMRC.

The merger with the Pharmacy College has been a real success story for Monash University.

Although the growth of Monash from a single campus university based at Clayton has been controversial and challenging, each campus is developing in its own way. They all contribute to a university which is unique in Australia in being able on the one hand to compete at the highest levels of international research and on the other to engage with regional communities and to provide opportunities for students who have lacked educational and socio-economic advantages to access a world-class university. Life would have been simpler if Monash had remained a single campus university, but it would have been likely to become a pale imitation of the University of Melbourne rather than the complex and exciting place it is today.

Not all my successors or future councils will share this view, as shown by the recent decision that the Gippsland campus would merge with the University of Ballarat to form a new institution, Federation University.

Chapter 25

MONASH UNIVERSITY MALAYSIA, SUNWAY CAMPUS

The concept of an international campus for Monash University was first conceived under Mal Logan in the early 1990s. Various sites and business models were considered. Singapore was a possibility, but eventually it was decided that Malaysia provided more opportunity in the long term. Despite some tensions between Malaysia and Australia at the time, Malaysia was seen as a country of great potential which had a need for more educational opportunities for students who were not Malays or 'Bumiputras'. The Malaysian government had overt policies setting quotas in tertiary institutions for Malays, Chinese Malaysians and Indian Malaysians, favouring Malays over the other ethnic groups. Many well-qualified ethnic Chinese and Indian Malaysians were therefore unable to access the best Malaysian universities. In many cases, the parents or other relatives of the students had been educated in Australian universities, often under the Colombo Plan scheme which provided subsidised places in Australian universities to students from South-East Asia from the late 1950s to the mid-1980s, when full fees were introduced for international students. Australian universities had a high profile and reputation in Malaysia as a result. Monash had been one of the most active universities in admitting students from Malaysia.

An essential part of the plan to establish a campus in Malaysia was a partnership with the Sunway Group, a large business conglomerate. The Sunway Group had started as a tin miner under the entrepreneurial leadership of its executive chairman, Tan Sri Jeffrey Cheah. With the collapse of that industry in the 1980s it had moved into construction and property development and had become the owner of holiday resorts, a shopping centre

CHAPTER 25

and hospital along with other lines of business. Its centrepiece was Bandar Sunway, a new town created in Petaling Jaya about 15 km from the centre of Kuala Lumpur. Bandar Sunway had been created by converting the tin mine into a hotel modelled on Sun City in South Africa, a large multistorey shopping centre complete with ice rink, a huge resort playground complete with artificial beaches and surf waves, many apartment blocks, a modern hospital, business offices and Sunway College.

After 'near death' experiences for the Sunway Group in the Asian financial crisis, the Malaysian campus of Monash was opened at Sunway in 1998. Initially, it was housed in inadequate facilities behind Sunway College. It was majority owned by the Sunway Health and Education Trust with Monash University responsible for the academic standards and for awarding the degrees. Monash did not have a financial investment in the infrastructure, and it received a royalty payment based on turnover. Initial schools included business and economics, arts, IT, engineering and science.

By the time I started as vice-chancellor in 2003, the campus had grown to about 2000 students. The pro vice-chancellor and head of campus was Professor Merilyn Liddell, whose original discipline was medicine (general practice). She was totally committed to the task of building the campus and believed that it was very important that a medical school was added. Clearly, the construction of a purpose-built new campus was also a priority.

My first visit to the Sunway campus was shortly after I started at Monash in September 2003. Graduations were being conducted at Sunway and in Singapore. A large formal dinner was hosted by Jeffrey and attended by many Monash alumni and distinguished Malaysian business people, bureaucrats and some politicians. I gave a speech in which I pointed out that this was a wonderful example of a mutually respectful way for a university to establish a foreign campus, in association with a trusted local partner that shared a commitment to the highest quality education and research.

Jeffrey Cheah invited us to his lavish home where we were entertained most generously. The evening included a singing performance by his formidable wife Susan. During this most pleasant evening, Jeffrey took me aside and told me how much he would value Monash establishing a medical school at the campus. Knowing Merilyn's enthusiasm for this, I made a commitment to Jeffrey that we would go ahead with this.

An important consideration in establishing the medical school was that we should gain accreditation for it by the AMC. This would require a reversal of policy by the council. When I was the chair of the accreditation committee of the AMC a decade earlier, the council had resolved, with my support, that it would not accredit off-shore campuses, even if they were campuses of Australian medical schools. This had been in response to an inquiry by the dean of medicine at Monash at that time, Bob Porter, and related to a plan to establish a partnership arrangement with a new medical school at Ipoh. Monash withdrew from the proposed scheme with some loss of face.

The AMC was initially reluctant to reverse this policy, and I and Ed Byrne, the dean of the Faculty of Medicine, Nursing and Health Sciences, had to appear before the council and use all our persuasive powers to encourage it to reverse the decision that I had been partly responsible for some years before. Eventually they agreed to do so, given that in this case Monash was entirely responsible for the academic standards of the degree. The graduates would be awarded the same degree as their Australian counterparts and their Malaysian colleagues who enrolled through the Australian arm of the medical school, and they would spend some of their time in Australia. The decision by the AMC to undertake the accreditation process was a critical one because it would ensure the standing of the new medical school and the transportability of the qualification. It did mean, however, that there could be no compromise on quality. Good staff would need to be recruited, first-rate facilities would be required and a research profile would have to be established if the rigorous standards of the AMC were to be met. Daunting though these requirements were, they were totally consistent with our ambitions for the school. To its credit, the board of Monash University Malaysia which comprised a majority of Sunway appointees did not resile from making the substantial financial commitment required.

We were fortunate in being able to persuade Anuar Zaini to come back from retirement to take up the post of head of school. A fellow endocrinologist, Anuar, had been the dean of medicine at the University of Malaya at the time I was dean at Melbourne, and we had become acquainted then. He later became vice-chancellor of the university. He was still relatively young and he had a young baby with his second wife, whom he had married after his first wife's premature death; he was ready to re-engage with academia with enthusiasm.

CHAPTER 25

Anuar recruited another old colleague of mine, Khalid Kadir, as professor of medicine and the research of the school received a great boost with the recruitment from Japan of a distinguished neuroscientist, Ishwar Parhar. The first students spent their first two years in Australia while facilities at the new campus were being completed and then returned to complete their clinical years at the Sultanah Aminah Hospital in Johor Bahru, where facilities for a clinical school had been built after considerable and protracted negotiations with the Malaysian authorities.

Monash Council decided to honour the key role played by Jeffrey Cheah in the establishment of the Sunway campus of Monash University and particularly the medical school by naming the medical school the Tan Sri Jeffrey Cheah School of Medicine.

The medical school was duly accredited by the AMC with glowing praise for what had been achieved and the quality of the educational experience of the students. Jeffrey Cheah and the Board of Monash University Malaysia were delighted and the success of the school was a credit to Merilyn Liddell, Anuar Zaini, the newly recruited local staff and the faculty from the medical school at Clayton who were tireless in their support for the school. Chris Browne played a particularly significant role.

Sunway completed a purpose-built new campus for the university in 2007. It was opened with great fanfare by Deputy Prime Minister Najib Razak (now the Malaysian prime minister). It provided modern, spacious facilities and accommodated the rapidly expanding research activity. The campus now has over 6000 students and is going from strength to strength. Professor Helen Bartlett has recently taken over as pro vice-chancellor from Robin Pollard.

The CEO of the Health and Education Trust of the Sunway Group, Lee Weng Keng, and the executive director of Monash University Malaysia campus, Phang Koon Tuck, were a pleasure to deal with and always conducted their dealings with us with the highest integrity.

I particularly acknowledge the commitment of Tan Sri Jeffrey Cheah to the campus. He was responsible for the foundation of Sunway College which initially provided feeder foundation programs to Monash University in Australia and to a number of other universities and then offered its own degrees as Sunway University College before becoming a full university. Although there was sometimes a potential for conflict of interest, Jeffrey Cheah emphasised that Monash was aiming to establish a leading research intensive university in Malaysia compared with the less lofty ambitions of Sunway University. Jeffrey was always extremely hospitable to Caroline and me, and we could tell when things were going well by which of his stable of Rolls Royces or Bentleys drove us to the airport.

Overall, although not without tensions and stresses at times, the Monash University Malaysia campus at Sunway has been a great success and has helped to strengthen ties between Australia and Malaysia. Jeffrey Cheah's part in this was recognised by the Australian government with an honorary Officer of the Order of Australia award, which was conferred by the then prime minister, Kevin Rudd, during a visit to Malaysia in 2008.

I have an ongoing relationship with Jeffrey Cheah as a trustee of the Jeffrey Cheah Foundation, which is charged with delivering philanthropy for educational purposes.

Chapter 26

MONASH SOUTH AFRICA

When I started at Monash, one of the most urgent and unresolved issues was the future of the campus in South Africa. David Robinson had persuaded the council to take the visionary but risky step of establishing a campus in Roodepoort about 30 km northwest of the centre of Johannesburg. Unlike in Malaysia, there was no partner to share the risk. At that time, the 100 hectares the university purchased for the campus was on the rural outskirts of the city, close to a large, poverty-stricken squatter township known as Zandspruit. The initial vision for the campus was that it should quickly become self-sufficient, repay the loan to Monash Australia and become a profitable activity for the university.

The first three years of the campus were fraught. Far from moving towards self-sufficiency, the annual deficit was growing. Student numbers were low, with only about 350 students in 2003 against a projected 760 at that time. The annual operating deficit was about AUS$12 million, and in straitened financial times, there was enormous antipathy to the campus by staff and students at Monash in Australia. In South Africa, although the government had initially been supportive, the current minister for education, Kader Asmal, a feisty Irish-educated Indian African, was opposed to foreign universities establishing campuses in South Africa and was making life difficult for John Anderson, the pro vice-chancellor in charge of the campus. I felt that it was likely that I would have to recommend to council that the campus should be closed. However, I recognised that this was not a step that I should take lightly, given the considerable efforts by many staff to get the campus to its current state, the commitment of the staff and students who had shown sufficient faith in the campus to work or enrol there and the huge reputational damage the university would suffer if it were to close the campus. Was it really serious about being a 'global university'?

The first graduation of twenty-one students was due to be held late in 2003 and I had my first chance to see the campus. I was enormously impressed by what had been achieved. The campus was in a stunning location on rolling hills on the outskirts of town. The property itself was impressive with an upper part that was suitable for developments and playing fields and a lower part, more wooded and with a creek, which would be a buffer against the rapidly encroaching suburbia. The campus buildings themselves were architecturally striking, with their Mediterranean style and uniformity. Student accommodation was excellent and teaching facilities modern. The staff, most of whom had been recruited locally, appeared committed and enthusiastic. Most impressive of all were the students – 75 per cent were African, 5 per cent or so Indian and around 20 per cent white. This reflected the ethnic diversity of the country. Many of the African students came from neighbouring countries such as Botswana, Zimbabwe, Kenya, Uganda and Swaziland, some supported by government or Monash scholarships, others with private funds. Many of the students were enrolled in the foundation studies program, which provided the educational foundation to commence a degree in the three discipline areas on offer – arts, business and economics, and information technology. About 15 per cent of the students were receiving bursaries from Monash.

The board of Monash South Africa was chaired by Paul Ramler, the deputy chancellor of Monash University. He was passionately committed to the campus and with the help of the pro vice-chancellor had assembled a most impressive board which at that time included Max Maisela, the head of the government superannuation fund and highly regarded by the ANC and Shirley Zinn, who was head of human resources at one of the large banks.

At the graduation ceremony, I met the high commissioner for Australia, Ian Wilcock. Ian had completed a postgraduate teaching degree at Monash and was an enthusiastic supporter of the campus. He said in his speech that he thought that the campus was the most important thing Australia was doing in South Africa at the time – perhaps a little hyperbolic in the light of the fledgling state of the campus.

I returned from South Africa convinced that it would be a significant betrayal of those who had worked so hard to get the campus established and of the staff and students who had committed to it. I also considered

CHAPTER 26

that the African continent was an area of enormous potential. As a country rich in resources with 800 million people and immense ethnic and cultural diversity, it would inevitably be a key player in the world in the future. There were obviously significant issues of governance, poverty and conflict for the continent to overcome, but I could see great advantages for Monash to become embedded in the continent through its South African campus and to be part of the education of many future leaders of sub-Saharan African countries. The research opportunities would be immense.

To achieve this potential would require considerable commitment by council and the whole Monash community.

First, I thought it was essential for us to clarify why we were in Africa. This was not a financial investment. It did not make financial sense for us to invest so much capital into such a risky venture with such uncertain returns. One could also argue about the morality of an Australian university making a net profit from education in a continent such as Africa which was very much in development mode. This had to be considered a strategic investment with returns to Monash that we could evaluate against our core values of excellence in education and research and a wish to have an international focus. If it were to be considered a strategic rather than a financial investment, Monash in Australia should not be placing commercial rates of interest on the loans to Monash South Africa. We did not do this when we were starting new programs such as architecture or building new buildings for specific disciplines – costs of such initiatives were shared by the university as a whole. By taking away the interest charges, there was at least a conceivable chance that the campus could eventually not only break even financially but repay the investment from Australia.

I also asked council to commit to the principle that Monash University would not repatriate net profit from the campus to Australia but would rather, when this happy opportunity presented, reinvest in education and research in Africa. The council agreed to this principle, which went a considerable way to altering the attitude of the South African politicians and bureaucrats to the campus.

It was still necessary to persuade council and the senior management of Monash that the campus was viable. It seemed to me that the best way to do this would be to employ an external consultant with experience in company strategy and financial analysis and planning. Some knowledge of higher education particularly in an international environment would also be very helpful. I thought that David Gilmour, an ex-partner in the Boston Consulting Group, with whom I had become acquainted in his role as a board member of the Australian International Health Institute of the Faculty of Medicine, Dentistry and Health Sciences at the University of Melbourne, would be ideal. This decision was endorsed by council and David agreed to undertake the task.

His report was highly influential. Essentially, he considered that the campus had the potential to be 'a jewel in the crown' for Monash. He advised increasing fees to make the campus viable and projected numbers and financial performance data which would see the campus break-even in an operational sense in about eight years' time, or in 2011.

On that basis, council decided to continue with the campus. Numbers of students increased although there was quite a dependence on the fragile, government-sponsored student intake from Botswana. The attitude of the South African government and the other universities remained unwelcoming and the campus was not officially recognised as a university in its own right. This had an impact on its standing but no direct impact on its function, as Monash University was awarding its own degrees which were recognised in South Africa.

The pro vice-chancellor, John Anderson, and I went on a tour visiting a number of the leading universities including the University of Capetown, Stellenbosch, Witwatersrand and Pretoria. Although warmly received, it was clear that the senior management of these universities remained confused by why we were there and I suspect were a little sceptical of our commitment to quality, collaboration and research and our lack of a profit motive.

We also visited the University of Botswana. During a gap in our program we made a brief visit to a small and somewhat rundown game park in the centre of Gaborone. We took a wrong turn and ended up in a rubbish dump. I could not help speculating that this might be a metaphor for the fate of Monash South Africa!

John Anderson and his colleagues had done a great job establishing the campus against considerable odds, but it was now time to consider appointing a head of campus who could more easily win the confidence of the government and the other universities.

After an extensive search, we offered the position to Professor Tyrone Pretorius. Tyrone was the deputy vice-chancellor (academic) of the University

CHAPTER 26

of the Western Cape, a quality university which had catered initially for the Cape's coloured community under the apartheid regime. Tyrone had grown up in poor circumstances with his family resettled from the centre of Cape Town to newly built, crowded apartments out of town. He was a psychologist and had two PhDs, the second earned while he was dean of health sciences at Western Cape to demonstrate to his staff that it was possible to do research as well as teach and have administrative responsibilities. Tyrone had impeccable 'struggle credentials' from the apartheid era. While a student at Western Cape, he would be imprisoned when he went to visit his mother's village during vacations so that he would not cause disruptions in the village. Tyrone is a private individual and these stories from his past only emerged gradually as we grew to know him better.

Tyrone is an inspiring orator. He is very well-connected with senior members of the ANC and with the senior public servants and his presence has been critical to the progress of the campus. Kgalema Motlanthe, the former vice-president of the Republic of South Africa (and president for a short time after the resignation of Thabo Mbeki), showed his confidence in the campus by sending his son there and Tyrone's friendship with Kgalema Motlanthe led to a greater recognition of the campus by the government and visits to the campus by ministers.

Following the Gilmour report, student numbers grew rapidly and new buildings, including additional student residences, were completed. The budget deficit did not decline as quickly as the Gilmour scenarios had predicted, indicating the need to increase fees. At one stage it looked as though 'break-even' would not occur till about 2016, but with the increases in fees agreed to by the board, the budget was almost neutral in 2013. The loan from Monash in Australia could then be gradually repaid, although new partnership arrangements with a private provider have recently altered the financial aspects.

Research collaborations, particularly involving water management, traffic accidents and the humanities, have been developed with other universities and with government authorities. A School of Health Sciences has been added. There are now almost 3000 students from all over sub-Saharan Africa. The students are inspiring and have started a volunteer program teaching numeracy and literacy to young people from the Zandspruit squatter camp each Saturday. There is active exchange of students between the South African, Malaysian and Australian campuses.

The campus has provided a unique opportunity for Australian staff and students who have visited and worked there to build relations with South Africans and to understand the complex problems and appreciate the huge potential of Africa.

An example of the special opportunities afforded by the campus came when our board member Max Maisela invited us to lunch at his house during one of our visits. A small contingent went along, including John Anderson, a Zimbabwean graduate from Monash in Australia who was working at the campus, and Gill Palmer, the dean of the Faculty of Business and Economics. A fellow guest was the foreign minister of South Africa, Dr Nkosazana Dlamini-Zuma and the former wife of the current president of South Africa, Jacob Zuma. She was a feisty woman who spent much of the time in a diatribe against Australia in general, and the Howard government in particular, for what she saw as its gratuitous interference in South African affairs in criticising the government's lack of strong action against the Mugabe regime in Zimbabwe with its evident infringement of human rights. I was tempted to say that without the 'gratuitous interference' of Australia and other countries in South Africa's affairs in the 60s, 70s and 80s, South Africa would be likely still to be suffering under the apartheid regime, but I held my tongue.

At the time, our high commissioner to South Africa, Ian Wilcock, had been unable to get an audience with Dr Dlamini-Zuma, indicating the 'privileged' position we were in. We were not able to alter the minister's views about the Australian government, but we trust that we made her more aware of our campus and why we were there and the positive impact it could have on education, research and collaboration between our countries.

Despite the progress, the campus remains controversial. It was a courageous decision to establish it, and it has required an enormous effort and commitment by many people to build it to its present size. It has had a positive impact on many students, and its graduates will have a major impact on the African continent. Having a significant number of leaders in politics, business, public service and other areas educated at Monash with Monash values and links to Australia will be of great benefit to Australia just as the Colombo plan was helpful in building relations between South-East Asia and Australia.

Overall, despite the questionable business plan and the controversial initial decision to establish the campus, its progress should be a source of immense pride to all at Monash who have been part of it. Political uncertainties remain in South Africa and there will likely be further challenges for the campus, but its establishment and progress have been remarkable achievements.

Chapter 27

MONASH UNIVERSITY IN EUROPE

When I started at Monash in September 2003, Monash had established two centres in Europe. The motivation behind the two centres was different and their subsequent fate has reflected this.

The Prato Centre was driven by the academic vision of a medieval historian, Professor Bill Kent. He felt that a physical presence for Monash in the heart of Italy would be a wonderful base for academics and students to study the art and history of the renaissance and beyond. Bill had a particular interest in Florentine history and had been taking groups of students there.

With the support of the Europe Steering Group, chaired by the dean of the Faculty of Law, Stephen Parker, possible sites were explored. In the end, the Palazzo Vai, an eighteenth-century palace in the centre of Prato was selected. Prato was about twenty kilometres from Florence and although its industrial outskirts are most uninviting, it has a well-preserved historical centre within city walls. The local authorities were encouraging and much of the palace was leased by Monash. It was fitted out with the help of a generous donation from Rino and Diana Grollo in late 1999.

The Prato Centre has been very successful as a site for teaching in a number of courses and for holding international conferences bringing together European and North American experts to an extent that is very difficult to replicate in Australia. Students love going there and it has increased the appeal of Monash to students.

Along with the obvious history and fine arts classes, some other faculties have found the centre to be very useful. International business and finance courses are conducted there and some lecturers come from London and other parts of Europe. The law faculty has collaborated with a number of universities in Europe and North America to bring students and faculty from multiple law schools together in a great example of true international education. Academics use Prato as a base to extend their research in European history, arts and other disciplines.

A second European centre was opened in 2002. Monash, under David Robinson, had developed a strong relationship with King's College London, the principal of which was an Australian, Arthur Lucas. King's College hosted the Menzies Centre which was supported in part by the Australian government. Robinson and Lucas, supported by the council of Monash had decided to establish a centre for Monash in a small building at Aldwych adjacent to Australia House. The idea was that this would be the base for developing a deep relationship between Monash and King's College with staff and student exchange and collaborative research and that the office would serve not only to expedite this but to serve as a base for Monash in the UK. Prospective students could gain information and make arrangements to enrol for an exchange, an undergraduate or graduate course or for a PhD at Monash in Australia. Merran Evans, a pro vice-chancellor at Monash was seconded to run the centre initially, spending part of her year in London and part in Melbourne.

The opening of the centre was fraught. David Robinson had just arrived in London to officiate when the 'plagiarism' scandal broke and he was rapidly recalled by the chancellor, Jerry Ellis, and took a return flight back to Melbourne before the opening. Deputy chancellor June Hearn then proceeded with the opening formalities with Monash receiving more publicity than it had bargained for.

Despite all the efforts of Merran and, later, Graeme Davison, who was seconded for a period to run the centre, when Arthur Lucas retired it lost momentum. There were some valuable exchanges at all levels, but the level of engagement never reached the heights that were envisaged.

When the Monash office was moved to the interstices at King's so that its previous site could be used by King's to sell memorabilia, we realised that the substance of the agreement with King's was not sufficient to justify the considerable expense of the centre so we withdrew from it.

My successor as vice-chancellor, Ed Byrne, has recently taken up the appointment as principal of King's, replacing Rick Trainor. Perhaps this will reignite the partnership.

The lesson from the London experience is that it is difficult to orchestrate partnerships from the top and that real commitment by the partners is

CHAPTER 27

required. This needs to involve funding initiatives that provide sufficient incentives for researchers and students to choose to collaborate with or to undertake exchanges at the partner institution so that real relationships can be built. Funded PhD and postdoctoral scholarships, jointly funded research positions and programs and fully funded exchange programs for students are required. There must be equal enthusiasm for the partnership on both sides.

Towards the end of my term, the deputy vice-chancellor (international), Stephanie Fahey, raised the possibility of a partnership between Monash and Warwick University. Warwick occupied a similar type of position in the UK to that of Monash in Australia. It was relatively young and had rapidly established itself as a leading research university ranked in top 10 of the Russell group of research intensive universities in the UK. Like Monash, it had a reputation for being innovative and engaged with industry. Most university ranking systems placed Monash and Warwick quite closely together. Like Monash, it had engaged in an active program of partnering with international universities.

I visited Warwick and was impressed not only by the quality of the university but also by the enthusiasm of the vice-chancellor, Nigel Thrift, and other senior members of staff to engage with Monash. We arranged for their pro vice-chancellor (research) and other senior staff to visit and agreed to develop the partnership further.

I am delighted that my successor, Ed Byrne, took this partnership to a much more mature form with joint appointments and jointly funded and supported research programs in major strategic areas. Rather than being based on MOUs and fine words, it has been welded together by a commitment by both parties to joint funding arrangements for people and programs.

Another initiative to build the research relationships with Europe in medical research commenced in the latter part of my time as vice-chancellor and has been more fully developed since. Nadia Rosenthal is a charismatic American who had been recruited from Harvard to head the Monterotondo (near Rome) outstation of the European Molecular Biology Laboratory (EMBL). EMBL consists of a consortium of twenty-one European countries jointly supporting basic biomedical research. It has its headquarters at a large biomedical research institute in Heidelberg in Germany which houses around 1200 researchers and PhD students, state-of-the-art research platform technologies and a newly built training centre. The outstation in Monterotondo concentrates on biology linking genetics with physiological and behavioural changes in mouse models of human disease. Outstations in Hamburg and Grenoble were associated with synchrotrons and concentrated on determining the structures of proteins, a key step in defining biological actions and in designing specific drug therapies. The outstation at Hinxton, near Cambridge in the UK, focused on bioinformatics and was known as the European Bioinformatics Institute (EBI). The EBI served as the major hub of bioinformatics in Europe.

Nadia met with Edwina Cornish who was invited to attend an EMBL Council meeting in Heidelberg, and on meeting the director general, Iain Mattaj, and the director of international programs, Silke Schumacher, the idea of Australia becoming an associate member of EMBL was conceived. This would consist of a network of partner laboratories centred around Monash University.

EMBL has a unique faculty structure. Outstanding early to mid-career scientists are recruited from around the world as group leaders. They are generously funded to support a moderate-sized research group with say a couple of post-doctoral researchers and a PhD student or two. The initial appointment is for five years and, subject to a satisfactory review, they are then appointed for a further four years, making a maximum period of appointment of nine years. Generally, they then readily find leadership positions in scientific institutes and universities around the world, most often in Europe. This model had been highly successful. EMBL is the leading medical research institute outside the United States as assessed by the number and impact of its research publications. Its alumni have had a major impact in the institutions to which they have been appointed. The model ensures that the most promising researchers can have secure, generous funding in their most productive period and also ensures continual renewal of talent and ideas.

Other elements of EMBL include highly sought-after PhD positions which include a high quality multidisciplinary PhD course and training programs open to scientists from member countries where latest techniques can be learnt. The core research platforms included a highly sophisticated advanced light microscopy unit where real-time images of changes in cell organelles and ion fluxes could be followed and analysed by the most powerful computer programs.

CHAPTER 27

Edwina Cornish, Nadia Rosenthal, Iain Mattaj and Silke Schumacher came up with a model for Australia to become an associate member. This would allow Australia to establish a hub and spoke network comprising the partner laboratory and housing group leaders and their groups appointed according to EMBL criteria with the five-year-plus-four-year structure. In addition, Australian PhD students could access the EMBL international PhD program if selected, and two group leader positions funded from Australia would be earmarked for Australia. They would return to an Australian institution after their first five years. A bioinformatics resource, which would house some of the more popular EBI databases, would be established.

After much negotiation, funding for the associate membership was secured from the four foundation participating universities (Monash, Queensland, WA and Sydney), CSIRO and the Australian government. A grant of AUS$8 million to establish two groups at Monash, to help establish the bioinformatics node at the University of Queensland and to cover administrative costs for the first five years was made by the Australian government with the enthusiastic support of the then minister for innovation, industry, science and technology, Kim Carr.

Australia was duly admitted as the first associate member of EMBL; Nadia Rosenthal was appointed as its inaugural scientific head and the partner groups were housed in the newly created Australian Regenerative Medicine Institute, which had been funded generously by the Victorian Bracks-Brumby government and was directed by Nadia. Two outstanding young scientists were appointed as group leaders and important databases were transferred to the EMBL Australia Bioinformatics Resource at the University of Queensland.

I was invited to chair the council of EMBL Australia on finishing at Monash and the other four Group of Eight universities accepted the invitation to join EMBL Australia. It is still a work in progress but with exciting PhD programs being developed, leadership of the Australian Bioinformatics Network and the recruitment of the former deputy director of EBI to define the mission and strategy of the Bioinformatics Resource Australia EMBL (BRAEMBL), EMBL Australia shows every sign of achieving the desired outcomes of better scientific collaboration with Europe and improving the international competitiveness of Australian biomedical research. Multiple group leaders in laboratories around Australia are being recruited.

Chapter 28

IITB-MONASH RESEARCH ACADEMY, INDIA

Monash University had taken the strategic decision to be a global university, not only in the traditional way by hosting international students and building research collaborations with universities and research groups in other countries but also by establishing a physical presence in a number of sites overseas. I was keen to maintain momentum in this area and in particular to investigate what we should do to build substantial and sustainable relationships based on a local presence with the 'Asian tigers', India and China.

Our campuses in Malaysia and South Africa were maturing to the stage where they were not only undergraduate teaching institutions but also research-intensive universities, contributing to research both relevant to their local environments and on a global scale. But this had been a resource-intensive process for Monash, in terms of time and human effort in the case of both campuses and financially for the South African campus. We could not afford to initiate another undergraduate campus in the next decade or so and it could be argued that this was not the best way to build the research links and collaboration that formed the major rationale for international campuses. Our experience had shown us that financial gain was not a realistic expectation of such ventures and indeed we had ruled this out in South Africa.

The real value of an international campus comes when it becomes research-intensive and able to attract the brightest researchers and students, form partnerships with local institutions and industry and access local sources of research funding because of its value to the local research effort and economy.

CHAPTER 28

In 2005, our dean of engineering, Tam Sridhar, approached me and suggested that we might explore establishing a research-intensive campus in India. This was totally consistent with the strategic approach that I thought was appropriate for our next international venture. India was a particularly appealing site for such an initiative. Education was hugely valued, English was widely spoken and there was a great need for more opportunities for the brightest students to undertake PhDs there. Both the Indian and Australian governments were seeking closer relations between the two countries.

Tam Sridhar was the ideal emissary to explore potential opportunities. He had completed his masters of engineering at the Indian Institute of Science in Bangalore before undertaking his PhD at Monash in the 1970s, and he had a very distinguished record in chemical engineering. He was a Sir John Monash Distinguished Professor, reflecting his research distinction and had been dean of engineering since 2003.

After his initial foray, he asked me to lead a delegation to investigate ways in which we might proceed to establish a research institute in India. Accompanying me and Tam were Edwina Cornish, the dean of science, Rob Norris and Megan Clark, the vice-president (technology) of BHP Billiton.

Tam had arranged an incredible visit. We started in Bangalore and visited the General Electric Research Laboratories and Infosys. General Electric was one of the first global companies to establish a major research effort in India, an initiative of its legendary CEO, Jack Welch. The rationale was that India was a relatively inexpensive place to establish a research institute, there was access to a large number of very bright and well-educated young people, and the IT infrastructure was quite well developed, with Bangalore rapidly developing as a global centre for IT innovation. Challenges, such as unreliable electricity supply and unclean water, could be addressed by in-house generators and water filters, and the difficulty with commuting could be addressed by a local accommodation compound.

The research laboratories established by General Electric were quite remarkable but no more so than the homegrown global IT giant Infosys. It was founded in 1981 by Narayana Murthy and six engineers with capital of US$250. It now has an annual turnover of more than US$7 billion, 153,000 employees and is one of the world's largest IT consulting and services companies. We met there an intern from Monash who had been selected as part of Infosys's global internship program.

On the way back from General Electric and Infosys to our hotel in Bangalore, we encountered one of the drawbacks of operating in India. Our driver decided that it would hasten our journey to leave the congested main part of the road to drive up a service road. Many cars, trucks and buses followed, filling the two lanes of the service road. The service road was separated from the main highway by a ditch about two-metres deep and one-metre wide. We then met two lanes of buses, trucks and cars coming the other way down the service road. Things ground to a halt. It seemed that there was no possible resolution. We would surely be there forever. But gradually over the next hour or so it was unpicked and a way through was found in the Indian way.

In Bangalore, we also visited the Indian Institute of Science and met with the legendary C. N. R. Rao. Rao is a world-renowned chemist, a much-decorated leader in the field of solid state and structural chemistry. He was the chair of the Scientific Advisory Council to the Prime Minister and was the lead author of a report advocating strict requirements for foreign educational institutions operating in India. We explored this with him and he made it clear that high-quality institutions such as Monash would not be affected by any proposed new regulations and would be welcomed in India.

We then visited the Indian Institute of Technology Bombay (IITB) in Mumbai. This highly regarded institution (despite its name it was really an engineering university with the power to award undergraduate and postgraduate degrees) was established in 1958 as the second of the prestigious IITs established under the subsequently adopted Institutes of Technology Act of 1961. They are the most prestigious engineering and technology education and research institutions in India and, with recent additions, now number sixteen. Almost 500,000 students compete annually for admission to the less than 10,000 new undergraduate places offered in the system. IITB has only 2200 undergraduate and 3500 postgraduate students. The students and most of the staff live on the campus which occupies 2.5 sq km in Powai, north of the CBD of Mumbai.

We spent some time meeting senior staff and particularly the director, Dr Ashok Misra, a distinguished polymer engineer. We spoke of possible models for partnership which would allow sufficient independence for a proposed joint institute with Monash to function separately, not

CHAPTER 28

constrained by the rigid and poorly remunerated employment conditions of IITB which made competition with the private sector for the best staff difficult.

It was clear that there were a number of very able scientists at IITB and a number of areas where there was a good match between research strengths at IITB and Monash. It was also clear that the physical facilities at IITB left a lot to be desired and the scientific equipment was often outdated. We felt that there was huge potential for a joint research institute if we could provide a new building and a governance structure that escaped from the rigid industrial relations and regulatory environment that was severely limiting the capacity of IITB to be internationally competitive at the highest level. Although initially Ashok Misra was nervous about creating an independent joint company structure with separate employment conditions, he recognised the benefits that could flow from it. His best research staff could hold joint appointments in IITB and the new institute and escape from the straitjacket that limited their salaries and flexibility to work with industry.

We agreed that to call any proposed institute by the name 'institute' would be confusing, given that IITB was already an institute. In view of the emphasis on PhD training, we thought that research academy might be appropriate.

In Mumbai we met with another of the leaders of science in India, M. M. Sharma. Like C. N. R. Rao, Sharma was a legend of Indian science, having been appointed professor of chemical engineering at the University of Bombay at the age of twenty-seven and later becoming director of the Institute of Chemical Technology in Mumbai. He was the first Indian engineer to be elected as a fellow of the Royal Society and he had been awarded the Leverhulme Medal of the Royal Society amongst many other prizes and awards. He was very supportive of our plans to form a joint research academy with IITB.

We then visited New Delhi. There we met with the secretary of the Ministry of Science and Technology. He was an enlightened bureaucrat who recognised the potential benefit of the proposed joint venture for Indian science and, although he warned us of the bureaucratic hurdles, he indicated that he thought that the Indian government would be supportive and might even provide some financial support.

Next we visited the minister for science and technology, the Honourable Kapil Sibal. He was an urbane and cultured individual who had trained as a lawyer, held a master's degree from Harvard and had published an anthology of poetry. He received us for morning tea in his home and, most impressively, had a prolonged and in-depth discussion with us without having a 'minder' present. We discussed the need for a variety of technology-based solutions for a number of India's challenges, including energy in the remote villages, pollution, clean water supplies and enough food to feed the burgeoning population. He was very supportive of the plan to establish a research academy in partnership with IITB as long as there was some focus on some of the problems confronting India. That was indeed the intention.

We then met with the Australian high commissioner in India, His Excellency John McCarthy, and his education counsellor, John Webb. They were both highly supportive of the proposal and promised all the support they could give.

After a number of additional functions and visits to research institutes in New Delhi, we had breakfast with Professor Ramesh Mashelkar. Ramesh is a charismatic engineer, who was about to retire from his post as director general of the Indian CSIR, the equivalent of our CSIRO. He was a friend of Tam and had had a long and distinguished record as a chemical engineer. He had been the first Indian to be the president of the UK-based Institution of Chemical Engineers and is also a former president of the Indian National Science Academy and an elected fellow of the Royal Society. He has received many international honours including honorary doctorates from twenty-six international universities. He is currently the president of India's National Innovation Foundation as well as the president of the Global Research Alliance. He has played a critical role in India's post-liberation science and technology policies. All this had been achieved despite growing up in poverty and walking to school barefoot.

Ramesh is a charming man and he was unrestrained in his enthusiasm for the project. He was later a Sir Louis Matheson Distinguished Professor visiting Monash in Australia on a number of occasions.

Following these visits, some of us proceeded to Dhaka in Bangladesh on a separate mission to discuss collaboration with the University of Dhaka. Bangladesh was experiencing a surge in interest in tertiary education which had led to a number of new private universities often run by entrepreneurs

CHAPTER 28

with doubtful academic credentials. During a visit to one such institution, there was an attempt to ambush me into signing an MOU between Monash and the private university which would have been seen as a great boost to the academic standing of this institution. After having been received with great ceremony, I was ushered into a hall full of dignitaries with a prepared MOU awaiting my signature and that of the president of the private university.

I quickly explained that we believed that MOUs should be driven from the bottom up. When we had evidence of collaboration between our researchers and scholars and those of the local university, we would then consider an MOU.

I extracted myself from that situation with some loss of dignity but without prejudicing the reputation of Monash University.

We were received with warm hospitality by the president of Bangladesh. The approach to his palace was complicated by street protests accompanying a long march from the countryside to Dhaka by supporters of an opposition MP in a highly charged political environment where two women were fighting for control of parliament. One of them, Sheikh Hasina, was the daughter of the assassinated Sheikh Mujibur Raman, credited with being the founder of modern Bangladesh.

Following the visit to Bangladesh, we proceeded to Kolkata for the launch of a joint symposium between Monash and the University of Calcutta on postcolonial writing. This was an excellent conference and led to exchanges of senior staff on study leave. Our visit to India finished at the University of Pune where our education faculty had established a collaboration. We were embarrassed when our driver got lost on the way to dinner with the vice-chancellor and a short drive that should have taken fifteen minutes took two and a quarter hours. Our driver lost his way when we were diverted from the most direct route by a procession celebrating some festival and the fact that he only spoke Bengali in a Marathi speaking community did not help.

Following this visit, I was convinced that the best way to develop a meaningful engagement with India was to go ahead with the formation of the joint venture with IITB to establish what became known as the IITB-Monash Research Academy. Megan Clark, the then vice-president (technology) of BHP Billiton, who had travelled and visited with us, was enthusiastically supportive and promised funding of approximately AUS$1.8 million over five years for scholarships. The dean of science, Rob Norris, was also won over, although not with quite the same level of enthusiasm as exhibited by Tam Sridhar, Edwina Cornish and me.

We persuaded council that they should commit AUS$10 million to underwrite the project, although funding would be sought from other sources, including Australian and Indian companies and the respective governments of the two countries.

We did not, at that time, appreciate the extent of the hurdles that would have to be overcome. The legal and regulatory environment in India was just as difficult to navigate as it is reputed to be. Loren Miller showed incredible perseverance and patience working with lawyers and accountants in both countries to finally establish the academy. Tam assembled a stunning board with luminaries from science and industry in both countries. Mohan Krishnamoorthy was initially seconded from CSIRO to seek Indian corporate funding and was ultimately recruited to be CEO of the academy.

The agreement to establish the academy was signed by Ashok Misra and me (in a six-hour visit to India) in Mumbai in 2007, in the presence of the Australian prime minister, John Howard, who was visiting India on a trade mission.

The formal commencement of the academy with recruitment of students was marked by a scientific symposium with over twenty researchers from Monash visiting Mumbai in November 2008. The official launch was performed by the high commissioner, John McCarthy, on 26 November. This was followed by a celebratory dinner. Later that night, I was awoken by a phone call from the high commissioner to say that a terrorist attack had taken place in Mumbai with many people being killed. I had another call later from Peter Marshall at Monash in Australia to ask if we were OK. I assured him we were and that we were staying in a hotel in Powai near the IITB, well away from the CBD and the Taj Hotel, which was the centre of the attacks. The terrorist attacks were followed by a siege, but none of our party was involved or at risk.

After all the work, I can now report that the academy is a great success, with over 100 extremely bright PhD students working on collaborative projects with supervisors from both the joint venture partners and substantial funding from the Indian government and some funding from the Australian government. Funds have also been raised from industry to support scholarships. The work of the academy is focused on water, clean energy, mining technology, simulation and life sciences, particularly stem cells. Our ambition to engage with India, its outstanding engineers, scientists and students, in a real way has been realised.

Chapter 29

MONASH UNIVERSITY IN CHINA

Just as our role in India presented a challenge and an opportunity, so too did our role in China. Many of our researchers were collaborating actively with researchers in China, and a close relationship had been established between our materials engineers and the Chinese Aluminium Company (CHALCO), a subsidiary of a state-owned enterprise. China was the source of more than one-third of our international students. Of course, with its burgeoning economy, China was already the dominant player in East Asia and, together with India, it had a trajectory that indicated that the balance of global international economic strength would progressively shift from the USA and Europe to Asia over the coming decades. We felt that we must strengthen our relationships with China to take full advantage of its amazing development and the emphasis that their leaders were placing on education and research.

It was soon clear to us that just as Monash was interested in China, so too were the Chinese interested in Monash. We had a close relationship with the Chinese consulate in Melbourne and I was also invited to address the Chinese embassy staff in Canberra on international activities of universities.

We were not keen, at that time, to establish a campus in China. We were fully focused on our Malaysian and South African campuses and our centre in Prato, and the research academy in India was soon to become a major preoccupation. However, we did not wish to wait too long before formalising some more substantive activities in China.

The Chinese consulate helped us determine the direction this should take, at least in the first instance. The consul general came to us and said that they would like Monash to have a special relationship with two Chinese universities. One was Sichuan University located in Chengdu in Sichuan Province in western China and the other was Shanghai Jiaotong University.

NEW TRICKS

Our deputy vice-chancellor (international), Stephanie Fahey, had already visited Sichuan University. She had established a cordial relationship with its president, Xie Heping, and recognised the potential value of a partnership with Sichuan University as it had a number of similarities with Monash.

In its present form it was a new institution. It had been formed in 2000 by the merger of the pre-existing Sichuan University with the Chengdu University of Science and Technology and the West China University of Medical Science. It had been designated as a high-level national comprehensive university under Project 985 and Project 211. It was intended to be the major university in western China, driving the academic and economic development of the region. Like Monash, it had around 60,000 students, two thirds of whom were undergraduates.

We were told by the consul general that China wished Monash to establish a close relationship with Sichuan University so that Sichuan could learn how Monash had become a world-class university in such a short period of time.

I led a delegation from Monash to China in 2007. Included in the delegation were Stephanie Fahey, senior representatives from the medical faculty, business and economics, science and the pro vice-chancellor in charge of the Monash Research Graduate School, Max King.

We were received with a great fanfare by Sichuan University. We were met at the airport, given a police escort through the city of Chengdu, and arrived at the university campus to be greeted by huge banners welcoming President Larkins and senior staff from Monash University. We were taken to a luxurious VIP guesthouse where we were to stay. We had a formal tree planting to mark the event and then the obligatory signing ceremony of the MOU.

We were taken on a tour of the newest of their three campuses. It was truly stunning. It occupied 400 hectares set in parkland with a central lake, not too far from the centre of the city. It had wonderful facilities, including a digital library that our universities would love to have. The university also had its own archaeological museum with ancient relics which were priceless. As it also was responsible among its many disciplines for training air traffic controllers, they showed us a wonderful 3D-simulation laboratory. It was clear that some first-class research was being conducted and that Sichuan University would be a worthy partner for Monash. We committed funding for some student scholarships and discussed ways we

CHAPTER 29

could take the collaboration forward. In particular, they were interested in management training for their deans and heads of colleges, and Stephanie Fahey organised a month-long program for thirty-two or so of their senior staff which was successfully conducted the following year (fully paid for by Sichuan University).

We were entertained at delightful banquets with the senior staff. Xie Heping was a generous and exuberant host with much toasting of each other with the potent sorghum spirit maotai. I am pleased to say that the Monash contingent did not disgrace themselves.

Our special host and guide in Chengdu was the vice-president (international affairs) Professor Shi Jian. He was a delightful, dignified man. Only gradually did his story emerge. During his youth he had been exiled to a remote Tibetan village for a number of years before being allowed to return to pursue his academic career. He did not appear to be bitter or resentful about this interlude in his life.

After two days in Chengdu, we were flown up to the adjoining Tibetan plateau. After a tourist trip in a minibus to a series of limestone ponds distributed down a mountainside from a peak of about 4000 m, we were taken to Jiuzhaigou International Study Center for Ecology, Environment and Sustainability which Sichuan University ran in partnership with the University of California, Arizona State University and Washington University. It was at the gateway to the Jiuzhaigou National Park, a stunningly beautiful and superbly maintained park with beautiful trees, a network of magnificent turquoise lakes and boardwalks and rustic tracks through the woods. There were also nine Tibetan villages in the park where the villagers continued to live a traditional life.

Our time in Chengdu concluded with Shi Jian escorting us to the Jinsha Museum which was constructed around an ancient archaeological site. There was also a panda breeding centre where pandas were apparently breeding happily in captivity in very pleasant surroundings.

The abiding impression from our visit to Sichuan was the sophistication of the university and the attention that had been paid to preserving archaeological treasures and natural beauty.

Our next stop was Shanghai Jiaotong University. Although the logic of the matching of Monash with Sichuan University was clear enough, the enthusiasm of the Chinese diplomats in Australia to team us up with Shanghai Jiaotong University was less clear. Shanghai Jiaotong was ranked number four in China. It had gained a significant international reputation by establishing the first internationally recognised and credible research ranking of universities. We thought that it might have its eye on the leading universities in the UK or the USA as special partners.

The rationale soon became evident when we visited the university. We were received once more with considerable fanfare, with banners and a delightful duck banquet hosted by the president. When we met the senior staff, the president said, rather disarmingly, that his university wanted to work with Monash, particularly in areas where they were less strong – the humanities and chemistry! Although he did not say as much, it was clear by the nature of his comments and the specificity with which he nominated the areas in which he wanted Monash's assistance that this was part of a well thought through strategy. They would try to get up to strength with Monash in their weak areas before exposing these to their higher profile partners, for example, Oxbridge and the Ivy League. Of course, we recognised the strategy, but we were not precious about it. We established a fruitful collaboration with Shanghai Jiaotong that extended beyond their nominated areas to medicine, business and economics and other areas.

I had a number of other visits to China, including signing a MOU with the Chinese Academy of Science and to attend a conference celebrating the partnership between Monash and Beijing University in establishing a stem cell centre of excellence.

On another occasion I also made a day trip to Beijing to sign and celebrate the partnership with CHALCO. This was performed with great ceremony in a guest house adjoining the guest house where the six power talks were being conducted trying to limit North Korea's development of long-range intercontinental ballistic missile capability. CHALCO provided support for our materials engineering and the outstanding research of Barry Muddle but the extent of the support never reached the level intimated by the suggestion of the formation of a CHALCO-funded research centre at Monash. Again, there was a suggestion of expediency about the support as CHALCO was at that time bidding for AUS$2 billion bauxite mine in North Queensland and was trying to establish its bona fides.

Towards the end of my time at Monash, we conducted the first of what was to become an annual graduation ceremony in Beijing. This reflected the importance we attached to building links with mainland China. We had traditionally conducted an annual graduation ceremony in Hong Kong, but

CHAPTER 29

given the demographics of our students, we decided to replace this with a ceremony in Beijing. As well as allowing our Chinese students to graduate in the presence of their parents, it also allowed us to invite prominent Chinese as well as Australian diplomats, including the ambassador, HE Geoff Raby. It was important for both prominent locals and senior Australian diplomats to be aware of what we were doing in China.

Not all our relations with China were as happy as those described above. Our Castan Centre for Human Rights Law headed by Sarah Joseph had invited the Dalai Lama to speak at Monash. I had a visit from the Chinese consul general telling me that the ambassador had instructed that I should not allow this. I explained that it would be a very sensitive issue for me to interfere in this way and, as a matter of principle, the organisers might well continue with the talk even if I tried to stop them. They would feel strongly that academic freedom was at stake. In any case, I said that I was not willing to try to stop the visit or the speech as I did not think it was appropriate for me to do so. This clearly upset the consul general, and I recognised that he had been instructed to stop the talk and his superiors would be very unhappy if he had totally failed in his mission. It could also have adverse effects on our welcome in China.

I decided to let the consul general have something positive to report back. I told him that I would not meet with the Dalai Lama or attend his talk. This was regarded as a sufficiently significant decision, given the hierarchical way of thinking in China. I rang Sarah to explain what had happened. As I had not been specifically programmed to attend the talk, it was not a real concession on my part but at least it enabled the consul general to maintain face and Monash to endure only a temporary loss of favour with our Chinese friends. The episode did, however, illustrate that despite the apparent warm relations there remained a gulf in the way that the Chinese hierarchy would choose to restrict freedom of expression and association and what is viewed as acceptable in our academic environment.

We were fully aware of the Chinese strategy of developing expertise in academic disciplines as quickly as possible by establishing partnerships, training programs and other links with our universities so that their institutions could compete at the highest level internationally. They were investing enormously in their universities and attracting Chinese researchers who had spent many years in the West to return to China. Whilst recognising that China would become more and more competitive in research and that our collaboration would help them to do this more quickly, we felt that it would be very much to our benefit to establish the closest links we could.

This policy has been taken to a new level by my successor Ed Byrne and the current council with the establishment of a joint postgraduate college with South Eastern University in Suzhou. The Chinese government is funding the resource and it will embed the links in much the same way as the IITB-Monash Research Academy has achieved in India.

Chapter 30

OTHER INTERNATIONAL ACTIVITIES OF MONASH UNIVERSITY

The international ambitions of Monash were not limited to Asia, Africa and Europe. Under David Robinson, there had been talk of establishing a centre in the US, but this had not been followed up. Stephanie Fahey, the deputy vice-chancellor (international), had built a relationship with Arizona State University, initially through a shared collaboration with Sichuan University. This led to a video link-up at one of our planning meetings but the marked decrease in state funding led to Arizona State, along with the other public universities in the USA, trying to cope with a budget crisis rather than putting energy into developing a relationship with a university on the other side of the globe.

Bob Charles, previously the federal member for Casey in Melbourne's south-west and a major force behind the Berwick campus of Monash, was appointed as the consul general in Chicago in 2005. As an alumnus of Purdue University, he saw potential for an academic partnership between Australian universities and American research-intensive universities in the Midwest. He encouraged the Group of Eight universities in particular to build such relationships and he prepared the ground by visits to the campuses. For Monash, his alma mater, Purdue, seemed the best fit. It is a multicampus university with its main campus in West Lafayette, Indiana. It is research-intensive with particular strength in engineering. Prospects for a special partnership were explored with a senior delegation from Purdue visiting Monash and vice versa. Despite considerable mutual admiration and strong support for the concept of a close partnership, other preoccupations of the two universities prevented this from developing into a significant relationship beyond the usual student exchange and researcher-led collaborations.

Many of our students benefit from placements in universities in North America and of course there are extensive collaborations between Monash researchers and those in American universities. I paid visits to a number of US universities and attended alumni functions. These activities paralleled those of other research-intensive Australian universities and, to date, Monash has not achieved a special positioning with respect to North America to rival its achievements in Malaysia, India, China, Africa and Europe. Similarly, although Monash has participated in the generous scholarship program offered by the Chilean government, the potential of linkages with South America has not been fully developed.

Monash has developed substantial interactions in the Middle East.

Following my appointment as vice-chancellor, but before I commenced my term at Monash, I was invited to address a fundraising gathering at Raheen, the stately mansion in Kew now owned by the Pratt family, for the Centre for the Study of Jewish Civilisation at Monash.

Monash University has a special relationship with the Jewish community of Melbourne. The inspirational figure after whom the university was named was a Jew. Its Caulfield campus is in the centre of the major residential location for Melbourne's Jewish community. Many prominent Jewish members of the Melbourne business and professional community have been educated at Monash and view it with pride and affection. Many are generous benefactors.

Along with support for other academic activities, the community had particularly supported the establishment of the Centre for the Study of Jewish Civilisation. Lee Liberman, the Pratt family, the Krongold family, the Gandel family and many others had been big supporters of the centre. It became a somewhat fraught issue as it was difficult to recruit a director of the centre. We were looking for a world-renowned scholar who could satisfy the donors' requirement for a high profile leader for the centre, the academics' requirement for high scholarly standards and the university's requirement for leadership and management skills. Fania Oz-Salzberger was indeed an inspirational and high-profile individual whom we did appoint to a chair, but she was only able to spend a small part of each year in Australia with the rest of her time in Israel at Haifa University. Although the centre has done some outstanding work, and has popular teaching courses, it has not yet quite achieved the profile the donors wished, and this has been the cause of some disappointment.

CHAPTER 30

In the process of seeking leadership for the centre and building academic relations with Israel, the dynamic and inspirational chair of the Australian Israel Chamber of Commerce, Leon Kempler, asked me to lead a trade mission to Israel in May 2006, dedicated to building academic links between our two countries. Several of our delegation were senior Monash staff.

It was an amazing experience. We were briefed on the political and economic climate in Israel by leading academics, politicians and bureaucrats and informed of the far-sighted policy by which the government provided seed funding for new technology development. This has led to the establishment of successful biotechnology, medical instrument and IT companies and also to the establishment of royalty and licence fee income to the research institutes and universities that exceeded that achieved anywhere else in the world.

The need for military and defence innovation, creative information technology scientists and a strong emphasis on medical research and medical instrumentation combined with imaginative government funding policies all combined to provide one of the best examples of the economic benefits from research and development.

We visited all seven research-intensive universities and had highly constructive discussions. Despite the generous and successful innovation fund that the government had sponsored in the nineties, there was considerable anxiety about substantial cuts to public funding of universities. Even in the light of the evident success of previous programs funding innovation in universities, in the face of financial pressures, the government was responding in the same short-sighted way as in other countries by reducing expenditure on education and research.

The visit was of course interesting in the geopolitical and historical sense as well. Most of the population went about their business ignoring the ever present threat of violence and war. Jerusalem is a fascinating city with its special meaning and religious monuments of the Muslim, Jewish and Christian faiths, including the various branches of Christianity. The Wailing Wall, the underground tunnels and the nearby remnants of Masada were all moving monuments of times past and important symbols for many today. A visit to the Yad Vashem Museum (the Holocaust Museum), in Jerusalem, was a particularly moving experience.

As in most sites of conflict in the world, the most noticeable feature of our visit was the lack of obvious tension between Muslim Israelis and Jewish

Israelis in the streets and in the education and medical institutions which we visited. Notably, many of the doctors and nurses and a large percentage of the patients at the Hadassah Hospital were Muslims and the deputy vice-chancellor (research) at Haifa University was Arab. The fundamentalist Jews who did not work and were supported by the state were a great concern to the average Israeli as were the fundamentalist Muslims to the average Muslim.

We learnt of an interesting collaboration when we visited the Weizmann Institute. Several Middle Eastern countries had agreed to fund jointly a synchrotron light source in Jordan to be known as SESAME. The collaborating countries included Jordan, Egypt, Palestine, Turkey, Pakistan, Cyprus, Iran and Israel. Given the Australian synchrotron at Monash, we were very interested in this development, not least because it demonstrated that mutual scientific benefit could circumvent political tensions which would seem to make such a level of collaboration inconceivable. It made the political tensions between Victoria and the commonwealth about the ongoing funding of further beamline development and operating costs of the Australian synchrotron seem trivial in the extreme. At the time of writing, the construction of SESAME is proceeding with its planned commencement of operations in 2015.

A particular highlight was a helicopter flight arranged for us by Lee Liberman from Haifa over the Jordan Valley and the Sea of Galilee to the Golan Heights. The Golan was heavily fortified and it was clear that it was highly strategic as it overlooked Syria and Lebanon. We then flew by helicopter to Jerusalem, where a lot of small fires burnt in celebration of a particular festival.

Our visit to the Golan was made even more significant a few weeks after our return when the war between Israel and Lebanon (Hezbollah) erupted with the Golan the centre of some of the most violent fighting.

The delegation visited the Ben-Gurion University of the Negev in Beer-Sheva and had interesting discussions with its senior administration on areas of common interest, including their program of research in desert studies and water supply. It was also interesting to learn of their efforts to extend educational opportunities to Bedouin young people and they now have over 500 Bedouin students, one half of them female.

We then had a memorable drive deep into the desert and celebrated my sixty-third birthday with dinner and music in a Bedouin tent deep in the Negev – quite a mystical experience.

CHAPTER 30

The trade mission to Israel led to the establishment of exchange agreements with the Israeli universities and research institutes. An indirect flow-on was the establishment by the president of Hadassah Australia, Ron Finkel, of the Australia Israel Medical Research Fund (AusIMed) to support clinical collaboration and bilateral research between the Hadassah Medical Center and high-level hospitals in Australia. Ron paid me the honour of making me a foundation patron of the fund.

Our interactions with the Middle East were not confined to Israel.

Shortly after I commenced as vice-chancellor, I received a three-man delegation from Iraq. The visit had been mediated by Dr Riadh al-Mahaidi, then a senior lecturer in engineering at Monash and now a professor at Swinburne University. He had emigrated from Iraq in the 1990s and was a personal acquaintance of one of the delegation, Dr Hussain al-Shahristani, then the president of the Iraq Academy of Science. Hussain had recently returned to Iraq following the downfall of the Saddam Hussein regime.

His story was inspirational.

After a period of education in Russia, Hussain had undertaken a BSc degree in chemical engineering at Imperial College in London and then MSc and PhD in nuclear chemistry at the University of Toronto. There he had met a Canadian woman, Bernice, who converted to Islam and married him. He returned to Iraq in 1970 to join Iraq's Atomic Energy Commission and worked on peaceful applications of nuclear technology.

When Saddam came to power in 1979, Hussain was told he must divert his nuclear technology to develop a nuclear weapon. He refused to do so and spoke out publicly against weapons of mass destruction and human rights violations. He was arrested, tortured for two weeks and then visited by Saddam's half brother. He was told that it was every Iraqi's duty to serve their country. Hussain agreed, but said that his idea of serving his country was different from that of Saddam.

He was put into solitary confinement in the notorious Abu Ghraib prison for the next eleven years, much of it in solitary confinement. The only reading material he was allowed was intermittent speeches by Saddam, and he was not allowed to write. He said that he was determined that although Saddam had captured his body, he would not allow him to capture his mind. He survived by playing mind games and, as a devout Muslim, praying.

In the confusion of a night-time bombing raid during the first Gulf War in 1991, he managed to steal the uniform and car of one of the prison's security officers and escaped across the border to Iran. He established the Iraqi Refugee Aid Council in 1995 to help the millions of refugees who had fled to Iran. He moved to London in 2000 where he continued his refugee aid work and was a vocal advocate for human rights in Iraq.

With the overthrow of Saddam by the 'Coalition of the Willing' led by the USA, he returned to Iraq and became the president of the Iraqi Academy of Science. He was drafted into the new government and helped with the framing of the new constitution. He became the oil minister in the Nouri al-Maliki administration and then deputy prime minister for energy affairs.

Monash was pleased to award him an honorary doctorate of laws in 2006. He captivated the graduating students with his address on the evening he received his award. His description of the events was self-deprecating and without bitterness and framed in the context that when offered a choice between right and wrong there is really no choice at all.

I was pleased to be one of many international sponsors of a nomination made for him for the Franklin D. Roosevelt Freedom from Fear Award, which was awarded in 2012.

Monash University had also developed a particular relationship with the United Arab Emirates (UAE). A member of the Faculty of Medicine Nursing and Health Sciences, Dr Nizar Farjou, had worked with the head of the School of Primary Care, Professor Leon Piterman, to develop a postgraduate diploma of general practice in the UAE. This enterprising activity led to Monash being well-known in the region.

One of the sheikhdoms of the UAE, Sharjah, was placing a particular emphasis on education as the way to guarantee its economic future. Unlike Abu Dhabi, Sharjah was not blessed with extensive oil and gas reserves. Dubai was a little better off, but realising that its supplies were limited to ten years or so, its leader, Sheikh Mohammed, had worked hard to make Dubai a trade and air transport hub and a site for the rich to holiday and spend their money. Emirates airline was one of his enterprises.

The leader of Sharjah, Sultan bin Mohammed Al-Qasimi, had been ruler since 1972, apart from a six-day period in 1987 during which an attempted coup involving his brother took place. He was an interesting and erudite individual, having initially received a bachelor's degree in agricultural engineering from the University of Cairo in 1971 and later PhDs with a distinction in history from Exeter University in 1985 and in political geography of the Gulf from Durham University in 1999. He is a noted

CHAPTER 30

historian and the author of a number of books. He was passionate about the environment and had created a huge reserve in the desert of Sharjah to protect the desert wildlife. Unlike some of the rulers in the region, he was liberal in his views and supported open dialogue with Western countries.

Sultan Qasimi had a vision for a tertiary education complex which he hoped would be the centre of learning in the Gulf. The complex consisted of two universities, the American University of Sharjah and the University of Sharjah. The ruler was the chair of the board of trustees of both universities. Although the American University of Sharjah was meant to be more Western and global in its orientation, the University of Sharjah was also intended to be global in its outlook and to engage fully with the rest of the world, although founded on the culture and history of the Islamic and Arabic world.

The board decided to establish schools of medicine, dentistry and pharmacy. After discussions, it asked Monash University to help the university to establish the schools of medicine and pharmacy, and the University of Adelaide was asked to help with the School of Dentistry after the University of Melbourne was unable to reach agreement with the University of Sharjah.

The partnership between Monash and the University of Sharjah was a very successful one, with good medical and pharmacy courses being established based on the Monash curricula. Despite some awkward discussions at times, the University of Sharjah agreed to most of Monash's proposals. Interestingly, this included establishing coeducational schools in contrast to the segregated classes in the rest of the university. The arrangement was financially very beneficial for Monash and served the University of Sharjah well.

The ruler and his entourage visited Monash University in Clayton. It was a warm and successful visit and he expressed his wish to work with Monash in the future. During his visit, he also met with the premier and asked the State of Victoria to establish a school founded on Western educational principles in Sharjah.

Following his visit, I was invited by the ruler to join the board of trustees of the University of Sharjah. I accepted, believing that building bridges to the Middle East would be very valuable for Monash. The board itself was very multinational, with senior academics from McMaster (the president Peter George), Exeter, Rochester and the American University of Beirut as well as local dignitaries. It was chaired by the ruler. A preliminary meeting of the academic committee chaired by the ruler's higher education adviser, a very sharp Egyptian named Amr, was held on the Saturday before the twice yearly meeting of the board of trustees. All the important issues on the board's agenda the next day would be discussed and a common position reached. The following day, the board meeting proper would be held, chaired by the ruler, and by and large, the earlier decisions of the academic committee were endorsed. The board meetings were routinely followed by a substantial banquet. The summer meetings were held in London where the ruler retreated for three months each year when the heat of Sharjah became too much for him to bear. He had a large estate near Gatwick Airport.

On the first of the board meetings after I became a member, a significant period was devoted to the ruler relating how the real estate developments by Sheikh Mohammed in adjoining Dubai were causing havoc with the coastal ecology of Sharjah. The artificial islands were interrupting the coastal currents and leading to the deposition of sludge on the coral reefs abutting Sharjah, causing the coral to die. He was very angry. The United Arab Emirates are united in name but far from united in their views. Indeed, the disparate wealth between Abu Dhabi on the one hand and Sharjah and the smaller emirates on the other (with Dubai in between) makes it very hard to achieve a common governance system for all the emirates, and local politics remains predominant in each emirate.

Sultan Qasimi proved to be a fascinating character, truly committed to education and the welfare of his people. He was apparently very popular with his people and no hint of the Arab Spring has affected Sharjah. As Sharjah had built up a dependence on business and trade for its economy, it was severely affected by the global financial crisis in 2008 and the promised funding for a chair of Islamic studies at Monash did not eventuate. Despite apparent financial difficulties for Sharjah, these had not apparently impacted too severely on the ruler's lifestyle. He had a passion for breeding Arabian horses and took us to a stunning horse show in Sharjah, where many of his horses were on display.

The international members of the board of trustees were thanked for their services and summarily told they were no longer required in 2010. It is to be hoped that this was a financial decision and did not reflect a desire by the ruler and his advisors to take a more narrow view about engaging with the rest of the world.

CHAPTER 30

I am pleased to say that Monash continues to have significant involvement with the Arab countries of the Middle East with licensing agreements relating to curricula with Abu Dhabi and Saudi Arabia.

Although there have been false steps along the way, the philosophy of my predecessors and particularly Mal Logan to make Monash a truly global university has led to some remarkable achievements and has placed Monash in a unique position amongst the world's leading universities. It has embedded relationships in South-East Asia, the Indian subcontinent, China, Africa, Europe and the Middle East. Collaboration and partnerships are built in a way that cannot be achieved by bilateral or multilateral agreements or 'student and researcher exchange' collaborations. Not only is this approach valuable for Monash, its staff and students, but it is also plays an important role in Australia's international positioning. The time, effort and money expended in this strategy should not be underestimated, but it has reaped rich rewards for Monash in terms of its global standing.

Chapter 31

UNIVERSITIES AUSTRALIA

The vice-chancellors of Australia's universities had long felt the need for some group therapy. The vice-chancellors of the six universities then existing formed the Australian Vice-Chancellors' Committee (AVCC) in 1920. Vice-chancellors, during this period, were part time and had limited powers. The real power resided with the professors and the professorial boards of the universities. I suspect that the AVCC was initially a social grouping rather than one that concerned itself with policy or advocacy to any large degree. Higher education at that time was accessed by only a tiny minority of the population and universities were not regarded as particularly important politically.

After the World War II, there was a gradual change in the attitude to universities. The creation of the Australian National University was a reflection of an initiative to promote research as a cornerstone of innovation and national pride. The vice-chancellors were becoming more vocal and responded to financial crises in the universities by publishing a document with the title 'A Crisis in Finances and Development of the Australian Universities', a forerunner of a number of similar pleas in the years to come. It recommended a national inquiry.

It took some time, but eventually the Menzies government established the Murray Committee, chaired by Sir Keith Murray, the chair of the Universities Grants Committee in the UK. The committee concluded that Australia's universities were understaffed and underfunded with weak honours and postgraduate schools. It recommended a greater role for the commonwealth in funding, including capital funding. The Menzies government accepted the recommendations and also introduced commonwealth scholarships, allowing bright students of limited means to attend university.

CHAPTER 31

Universities have been subjected to countless enquiries, policy changes and administrative changes ever since. The binary system of tertiary education with technical colleges and colleges of advanced education introduced in the 1960s was replaced by the unitary system following the Dawkins reforms of 1988 with amalgamations and reclassifications of many former colleges.

At times, universities have been seen as an appropriate target for increased government expenditure, notably by the Menzies government following the Murray review, the provision of free university education by the Whitlam government and the uncapping of student numbers by the Rudd government. More often, they have been seen as possible sources of savings for the government, notably with the introduction of a student contribution to the fees (the higher education contribution scheme or HECS) and full-fee places for international students by the Hawke government and the introduction of full-fee places for domestic students and the increase in HECS by the Howard government. Despite the Bradley and Lomax-Smith reviews, both recommending an increase in base funding of universities, the recent (2014) commonwealth budget proposes a 20 percent cut in university funding by the commonwealth, with deregulation of the student contribution.

In any event, far from being the erudite institutions functioning on the outer boundaries of society and affecting few as was the case before World War II, universities are now politically relevant and subjected to a morass of compliance and funding requirements which require constant and powerful advocacy from their vice-chancellors.

The AVCC had an image problem which reduced its ability to lobby effectively. The media regarded it as a club for overpaid vice-chancellors, allowing them to go on jaunts at the expense of their tax-payer funded universities. Media photographs of vice-chancellors riding camels on Cable Beach in Broome during the first AVCC meeting which I attended did not help to dispel this image. The annual universities meet parliament dinners were lavish affairs held at Parliament House in Canberra and reinforced the view of many politicians that universities were not underfunded and that their vice-chancellors were more interested in extravagant dinners than in the welfare of students at their universities.

The government regarded the AVCC as adversarial, always critical and whingeing about funding. In contrast to the politically sensitive nature of school funding, governments did not see it as politically valuable to give more government funding to universities. The AVCC had failed to convince the community or big business of the self-evident fact that universities were critical to the future of the country so governments were given no incentive to give priority to concerns of the universities as expressed by the AVCC.

Moreover, the universities themselves were finding it difficult to speak with a single voice. Factions had developed and groups of universities were finding it easier to find a common voice in groupings such as the Group of Eight, the Australian Technology Network and the Innovative Research Universities, and there was even an attempt to give a structure to the unaligned universities. Whatever political influence that universities might otherwise have had was considerably weakened by the divisions between them.

Some of my colleague vice-chancellors from the Group of Eight universities (the University of Adelaide, the Australian National University, the University of Melbourne, Monash University, the University of New South Wales, the University of Queensland, the University of Sydney and the University of Western Australia) tended to stay away from meetings of the AVCC. They felt that the well-resourced administrative structure of the Group of Eight, together with the obviously superior research performance of the Group of Eight universities (together they received about 75 per cent of total research funding and produced over 75 per cent of research outputs of the thirty-nine universities), would make them more effective advocates than the diverse and divided voices within the AVCC as a whole.

My view was a little different. Some of the Group of Eight vice-chancellors put great store in the evidence of superior research performance and the much larger budgets of their universities to persuade the politicians of the importance of acceding to their requests. But pragmatism suggested that regional universities in marginal electorates and some of the newer universities with campuses in outer suburban areas where many seats lay in the balance were more important politically. The connection between regional and outer suburban universities and the voters in the community was stronger than in the Group of Eight universities which were largely based close to the centres of large capital cities without any close links to the voting public.

There were important issues confronting the universities. The Howard government had targeted university funding to help fund a budget deficit when it came to power in 1996. The infamous 'Vanstone cuts' (named after

CHAPTER 31

Amanda Vanstone, the education minister at the time) led to a decade in which Australia was the only OECD country to decrease (in real terms) public funding of its universities. Full-fee domestic places, up to a maximum of 25 per cent of the quota of places, were introduced for undergraduate courses, and universities were encouraged to increase their intake of fee-paying international students. The universities were becoming increasingly overcrowded and new capital funding was minimal. Research funding was stagnant, although the Wills Review of health and medical research in 1998 did lead to a significant increase in funding in this area.

There were also difficulties for students from economically disadvantaged backgrounds accessing university. The student contributions through HECS had been substantially increased, leading to sizeable debts on graduation, although the enlightened repayment scheme contingent on income partially offset the impact of this. More importantly, the living expenses for students made it very difficult for poor students to attend university and those that did had to work often in demanding jobs which detracted from their ability to attend their university campuses.

As an elected member of the board of the AVCC and, from 2006, the deputy president to Gerard Sutton of Wollongong University, I had been engaged in advocacy for universities and their students from 2005. It was an interesting experience as many of the ministers in the Howard conservative government had entrenched views against universities. One senior minister described universities as the last refuge of socialists and student financial support as 'middle class welfare'. Another senior minister, whose portfolio was directly responsible for innovation and industry, when presented with arguments relating to the relatively low proportion of GDP spent on research and development and the underfunding of research in our universities, said that he 'didn't much care for statistics of that sort. I am only interested in the rate of growth of our GDP and that is going gangbusters so we must be doing something right'. The fact that the GDP was being driven by demand for our resources and a housing boom driven by increasing household debt and was not sustainable without new investment did not seem to concern him. The education minister was fond of responding to arguments for increased funding of universities by firstly saying how badly the universities were being managed and then describing the operating surpluses as profits, indicating that the universities were obviously receiving plenty of funding. She did not wish to acknowledge, despite having it pointed out to her, that the operating surpluses were required to fund new capital development and did not reflect a cash surplus.

Under the strong leadership of the vice-chancellor of Wollongong University, Gerard Sutton, the AVCC set out to improve its image and to become more effective. At the AGM of the AVCC in 2007, several substantial changes were made to the name and the constitution of the AVCC. It was to become Universities Australia, and its members would be the universities, not the vice-chancellors, although the new constitution clearly stated that the universities were to be represented on Universities Australia by their vice-chancellors as the chief executive officers of the universities. A separate council of chancellors was formed where the chancellors would meet twice per year and discuss matters of mutual interest relating to the governance of universities. A joint meeting with the vice-chancellors was planned annually.

The position of president of the AVCC was to be renamed the chair and the administrative head of the office of Universities Australia was to take more responsibility for public comment and advocacy and would assume the major role as the public face of Universities Australia. This was in recognition of the time constraints of the vice-chancellor elected to the chair position and the continuity provided by the CEO with a longer term of office than the president.

The long-serving CEO, John Mullarvey, a passionate advocate for universities, had achieved a great deal for universities. He was a key figure in establishing AARNET, the network allowing university campuses in Australia access to high speed internet, in bulk purchasing arrangements for universities, for negotiating arrangements, allowing universities to access and reproduce copyright written material at a fraction of the usual cost and through advocacy had been responsible for significant increases in university funding in the Nelson 'reforms' of 2003. John revelled in being a larger than life character, who was sometimes viewed as overly adversarial with departmental bureaucrats and the ministers' offices.

John resigned in 2007 and, after an extensive process, Professor Glenn Withers, an economist with the Australian National University who had previously held a number of government positions, was appointed as CEO. Tragically, John Mullarvey died of disseminated melanoma in 2009 at the age of fifty-eight.

I succeeded Gerard Sutton as chair of the newly constituted Universities Australia in January 2008. It was shortly after the election of the Rudd-

CHAPTER 31

Gillard Labor government. They had placed considerable emphasis on education during the election campaign.

It was an interesting experience. Vice-chancellors by and large are not a shy and retiring lot and most of them held strong views on the many issues confronting universities and how they should be addressed. I had the choice of trying to reach consensus on contentious issues where the vice-chancellors had widely differing views (for example, on deregulation of undergraduate fees) or leaving those issues alone for the individual groupings to argue their case and concentrating on those issues where there were common views. Central among these was the need for more financial support for economically disadvantaged students, more public funding for universities, a proper formula for calculating indexation of public funding and more funding for research. A research assessment exercise (RAE) was being planned by the Howard government based on the RAE in the UK. The model proposed was excessively demanding and included an assessment of the impact of research – for example, on industry, public policy or other demonstrable public good outcomes. The universities were divided on including impact and indeed on the value of a RAE at all. The RAE as proposed by the Howard government was abandoned when Rudd came to power, and the ARC was charged with establishing some other model. The ARC under the leadership of Margaret Sheil developed a program which became known as Excellence in Research Australia (ERA). These were hot issues during my time as chair of UA.

The ministers with whom I was most involved were the minister for education, Julia Gillard, who was also the deputy prime minister and the minister for innovation, industry, science and research, Kim Carr. Both at different times addressed the newly introduced Higher Education Conferences of Universities Australia and spoke passionately about their belief in the fundamental role of universities in the economic development of the country and in providing life-transforming opportunities for students. They spoke of their own experiences in that regard. Other influential Labor ministers shared their view including Lindsay Tanner and Craig Emerson and Kevin Rudd himself had made similar comments.

As with all politicians that I have had contact with, there were sensitivities verging on paranoia. As an example, one Wednesday shortly after I had taken up the role of chair of UA, I had a phone call from the head of Julia Gillard's office. He said in a stern voice that Julia did not like that bit in the Higher Education Supplement of the *Australian*. As I was not aware of anything I had said that he might have been referring to, I asked him to explain. He said it was the quotation from Glenn Withers as CEO of UA, where he said that he did not think that the current government was fully aware of the degree of neglect of funding of universities over the last decade. I said that this comment seemed to be directly critical of the Howard government, not of the newly installed one, but I had it pointed out to me that Julia Gillard prided herself on being across all the issues and did not like any implication that she was not. To emphasise the general displeasure, he concluded by saying that Kevin (Rudd) and Wayne (Swan) did not like it either!

Kim Carr was genuinely enthusiastic about the role of university research in innovation and introduced a number of schemes designed to enhance Australia's research capability. The National Collaborative Research Infrastructure Strategy had been introduced and included in an earlier Howard-Costello budget but was implemented by Carr, and there was also added Super Science funding. After the Cutler Review of innovation policy there was a plan to gradually increase the funds available to support unmet costs for research in universities although this has subsequently been stalled. Carr was a true friend of universities and research, but unfortunately he was on the wrong side in the leadership shenanigans that saw Gillard replace Rudd and ultimately resigned from the ministry completely after an earlier demotion.

On a casual meeting some months later, he predicted that 'we will be back' and this proved to be the case when Rudd replaced Gillard.

Gillard introduced a review of higher education chaired by Denise Bradley, formerly vice-chancellor of the University of South Australia. Among many recommendations was the need to increase participation, with a target of 40 per cent of twenty-five to thirty-four-year-olds holding a tertiary degree by 2020 as compared with the figure at the time of the review of 29 per cent. It was also recommended that 20 per cent of students in higher education should, by 2020, be from the lowest socio-economic quartile compared with the current figure of about 15 per cent. It was recommended that places should be offered to all qualified students, with students choosing where they would study, and with funding to follow the student. It was also recommended that base funding per student should be increased by 10 per cent and that a new regulatory agency should be established.

There was a recommendation about better-targeting student welfare support. UA was united in the view that more student support was required to allow economically disadvantaged students to attend university and not

CHAPTER 31

just a reallocation of the funds currently distributed as the government had decided. This was a controversial decision by the government. Part of our advocacy included meeting with bureaucrats from the department responsible for social services and welfare, and we experienced some of the attitudes which reflect the extent to which universities and the government are at cross purposes with respect to student support. The attitude expressed was that students smart enough to get to university would be smart enough to look after themselves and therefore did not require government support. This was contradictory to the attitude expressed by the minister for education (Gillard) and the department of Education, Employment and Workplace Relations which saw student financial support as necessary to achieve higher participation rates in higher education.

The recommendation to uncap the number of student places was introduced with many universities increasing their intake of students quite considerably, often with a commensurate lowering of entry requirements. This was predictably expensive for the government. Funding per student was not increased despite the recommendations of the Bradley Review and a subsequent review of base funding headed by the Honourable Dr Jane Lomax-Smith that there should be an immediate 10 per cent increase in the per capita base funding rate. The recommendation to form a new regulator which was known as the Tertiary Education Quality and Standards Authority (TEQSA) was adopted. A realistic rate of indexation of base funding was introduced to take effect from 2012, but like the plan to increase the funding of the indirect costs of research, this was interrupted with the budget constraints associated with trying to achieve a budget surplus and fund the recommendations of the Gonski Review of schools' funding.

The funding of major capital infrastructure for universities was also an active issue. Peter Costello, the treasurer in the Howard government, had established the Higher Education Endowment Fund (HEEF) with an initial allocation of AUS$5 billion from the budget surplus in 2006–07. It was intended that an allocation would be made from the fund annually by the minister following a competitive process on the advice of an expert committee. The fund would be maintained on a perpetual basis and expanded from future budget surpluses.

In the event, with the global financial crisis of 2008, most of the corpus of the now expanded and renamed Education Investment Fund was allocated to universities in the hope of stimulating economic activity by new capital development. As usual, there was almost no lead time before this huge splurge on capital funding, but the allocation did result in many fine capital projects being funded. The time required for design and preparation meant that, for the most part, the global financial crisis had been weathered by the time there were actually 'shovels in the ground'. Little of the Education Investment Fund remains and budget surpluses to replenish it seem a distant dream. So the idea of a perpetual fund for university capital development seems to have vanished.

At the time I finished as chair of Universities Australia in May 2009, things were looking pretty positive for university funding. Much of the disappointment lay in the future. When things get tough, university funding is an early target for governments. We still have not succeeded in convincing the community, and thus the politicians, of the absolutely critical role that top-class universities play in the economic and cultural health of the country. A wealthy country like Australia should make available to all who have the ability and wish to benefit from it the life-transforming opportunities that tertiary education confers.

As chair of Universities Australia, I was a member of the Prime Minister's Science, Engineering and Innovation Council. I had previously been a member of this council while chair of the National Health and Medical Research Council. I had met Kevin Rudd previously when he had attended a couple of dinners of the board of Universities Australia when he was the leader of the opposition. It was already apparent from those meetings that he had a razor-sharp mind and a natural instinct to demonstrate this to all around. He was also intent on arming himself with ammunition with which to attack the Howard government. Whenever reference was made in general terms to problems confronting the universities as a result of government decisions, he would ask for three specific examples.

As chair of PMSEIC, it was clear that he had a strong sense of the excitement and importance of being on the world stage. For example, at a meeting in early 2009, not long after the global financial crisis had erupted, he announced that he was expecting a call from Gordon Brown, then the prime minister of the UK at 10 a.m., and would have to leave for a few minutes, presumably after he had given the appropriate advice to the UK prime minster on how to deal with the crisis. He was very engaged by a presentation led by Fiona Stanley on Indigenous health. Not satisfied with the excellent summary given by Fiona, he then summarised in his own words and, in a slightly manic manner, announced the deliverables to which the government

CHAPTER 31

would commit. He was a man of high intelligence and huge energy whose thinking was a long way ahead of the ability of those around him and indeed his own ability to transfer his worthy intentions into successful actions.

My time on PMSEIC coincided with the release of the Cutler Review of Innovation in Australia. I led a presentation of aspects of that review and its findings to the council. The prime minister was clearly interested, and some of the recommendations of the review were subsequently implemented, although it is disappointing that this has been in a piecemeal fashion without a strategic long-term plan to improve the pipeline from basic research through to innovation and increased productivity. The implementation has been marked by interruptions driven by reversals caused by budget constraints and uncertainties associated with the demotion of Senator Kim Carr from cabinet and his dismissal from the innovation and industry portfolio. Subsequent rapid turnover of portfolios has seen five ministers responsible for innovation industry science and tertiary education over eighteen months. There is little wonder that there has been no coherent policy implementation.

I am pleased to say that despite a few difficult moments along the way, I left Universities Australia as a functional, effective organisation that was having a positive effect on public and political perceptions of universities. I delivered a National Press Club address emphasising the importance of universities to Australia's future and it seemed to be well received. The annual Higher Education symposia being mounted by UA were well attended and supported by politicians and the media. There was a higher level of trust between the different universities than had been apparent when I became chair. It is pleasing for two reasons that another Group of Eight vice-chancellor, Glyn Davis from the University of Melbourne, was elected as chair following a successful tenure by Peter Coaldrake of the Queensland University of Technology. The first reason is that it shows that he thought as I did that the role was important enough for him to take it on. The second reason was that it showed that the vice-chancellors of the rest of the universities had enough confidence in the Group of Eight to once more elect one of the Group of Eight vice-chancellors as their chair.

However great the differences between the universities in Australia, I am convinced that their cause is best served by having a collective voice advocating for the importance of their role to the future of the country and, for that matter, of the planet. Where there is no common voice, the subgroups can have their separate opinions, but for the big issues, there is great strength if all can speak with a single voice.

Chapter 32

FAREWELL TO MONASH

My appointment to Monash was due to finish at the end of 2008. Because of my role with Universities Australia, I requested an extra six months and this was graciously granted by the council of Monash University with my tenure set to end on Friday 3 July.

My last six months were as hectic as any during my time at Monash. As well as the usual visit for the annual graduation ceremony at Monash South Africa in February, a further visit to the campus was planned to launch a joint research initiative involving the Monash University Accident Research Centre relating to road accidents in South Africa, a huge public health problem. This visit was associated with a colourful and moving farewell. I was given a framed aerial photograph of the much expanded campus labelled 'Your African Footprint'. In the African style, there was much singing and dancing and generous speeches.

A very brief visit to the Malaysian campus for a board meeting was marked by the gift of a Selangor pewter walking stick to mark my retirement. I have been pleased to be able to continue my association with the campus as Tan Sri Jeffrey Cheah asked me to be a trustee on his newly created Education Foundation.

Monash gave me a wonderful farewell dinner at the Melbourne Museum. The chancellor, Alan Finkel, the premier, John Brumby, and Edwina Cornish all said generous things about my time at Monash, and I had the opportunity to say what a wonderful experience and privilege it had been for me.

Many less formal farewells with individual faculties, the committee of deans, various campuses and other groups followed. The staff was due to give me a final farewell on my last day. Unfortunately, I had the second episode of an acute bacteraemia that led to me being in hospital for six days before that final farewell. I was allowed out of hospital just in time to attend.

CHAPTER 32

My time at Monash had come to an end. It had been an exhausting time with much travel, many difficult challenges and a huge personal workload. But it had also been an immensely rewarding time. Many people remarked that the university was at a low point in its history when I took over. It was recovering from the difficult situation associated with David Robinson's departure and there were still residual divisions in the university between those who had been supporters of David Robinson and those who had played a part in his forced resignation. Research performance had not kept up with the other Group of Eight universities and there were concerns about teaching quality and the ever-present concerns about the budget. The senior management team, like the rest of the university, was divided. Peter Darvall had done a great job while he was the interim vice-chancellor but without a definitive long-term role he had a limited ability to turn things around.

In many ways, it is easiest to take over an organisation when it is at a low ebb because it can only go upwards. All the ingredients were there for the university to continue its meteoric rise to be one of the world's best universities. By re-emphasising the importance of education and research, the staff felt once more that the university was on the move again, and they responded superbly. Gradually we were able to assemble a senior management team that was the equal of any in Australia and it was very rewarding to see all the objective parameters of success improve so markedly.

Edwina Cornish played a major role in building the research output by supporting good researchers already at the university and providing an environment that attracted stars from around the world. Stephen Parker and, later, Adam Shoemaker were responsible for instituting major improvements in education, including implementation of new technology, and Peter Marshall and David Pitt were responsible for administrative and financial oversight at a very professional level. Ron Fairchild launched a major fundraising campaign and was almost halfway towards a target of AUS$200 million by the time I left. Stephanie Fahey had developed the partnerships with Sichuan University and Warwick University and exciting initiatives in the Middle East.

John Brumby, initially as the minister for innovation and treasurer and later as the premier, had been enormously supportive, providing substantial funding for new initiatives and in providing the bulk of the funding for the Australian synchrotron located at Monash.

NEW TRICKS

I left Monash with a feeling of great affection for an institution that I had only really begun to know six years before. The ambition of the staff to really make a difference through education and research was refreshing, and the passion and enthusiasm of the students gave me immense confidence for the future. They will be equipped as we are not to deal with the immense challenges facing the world in the years to come.

I feel privileged to have played a small part in the history of this inspirational institution.

Chapter 33

LIFE AFTER MONASH

Caroline and I had a wonderful seven-week holiday in London, Wales, Provence and Tuscany after I finished at Monash.

I returned to a portfolio of activities that I had been asked to take on and which have provided me with a significant buffer against the risk of 'relevance deprivation syndrome'.

I had been asked by Daniel Andrews, then the minister for health, now the leader of the opposition in Victoria to chair the Parkville (now Victorian) Comprehensive Cancer Centre Joint Venture. This ambitious project was centred around the relocation of the Peter MacCallum Cancer Centre from East Melbourne to a triangular block, previously the site of the dental hospital which was adjacent to the Royal Melbourne Hospital and diagonally opposite the University of Melbourne. A new building was to be erected on the dental hospital site which would house the Peter MacCallum Cancer Centre, new laboratories for the University of Melbourne, new laboratories for the Melbourne Branch of the Ludwig Institute and the headquarters for the Victorian Cancer Centre Joint Venture offices. Across Grattan Street and joined by above ground walkways at two levels, three additional stories were to be added above the emergency department of the Royal Melbourne Hospital which would provide new facilities for cancer patients on that site. There would be a new intensive care unit, new operating theatres and of course the full range of radiotherapy, day care, pathology and imaging services spread between the two sites together with greatly expanded research laboratories. The new building project would cost over AUS$1.1 billion, with AUS$424 million each from the commonwealth and state governments, AUS$25m from the University of Melbourne, AUS$12.5m from the Ludwig Institute and the remaining funds to be raised by sale of assets at the East Melbourne site and by fundraising.

In addition to the building project, the relevant ministers and the department of health had decided on this major investment on the basis that a 'comprehensive cancer centre' as defined by the National Cancer Institute in the USA would be formed. This implied that there would be an integrated program involving cancer prevention, treatment, and research at basic, translational, clinical, population and health services levels and education programs involving all professional disciplines and public education. An incorporated joint venture, with the responsibility for implementing this program, was formed with a membership comprising the Peter MacCallum Cancer Centre, Melbourne Health, the Walter and Eliza Hall Institute, the University of Melbourne, the Royal Women's Hospital and the Ludwig Institute. The board was to be comprised of me as the independent chair, Dr George Morstyn as the independent deputy chair, the dean of the Faculty of Medicine, Dentistry and Health Sciences at the University of Melbourne and the chief executives of the other partners.

The politics of this were always going to be difficult as there had been a long history of tense relations between the Peter Mac and the Royal Melbourne. When Peter Mac was relocated from its original site in William Street in the late 1980s, many at the Royal Melbourne Hospital felt that it should be collocated with the Melbourne. Peter Mac feared that this might lead to its loss of identity and impair its ability to provide outstanding cancer care to its patients. After intense political lobbying, it was decided to relocate it to St Andrews Hospital in East Melbourne, a private hospital which was closing.

The board of the joint venture soon resolved to add the Royal Children's Hospital to the joint venture, given its geographic proximity and the need to integrate the care of its patients with Melbourne Health and Peter Mac to which many of them would ultimately be transferred. A little later, after quite intensive discussion, St Vincent's Hospital and Western Hospital were added as they had very close clinical and education links with Peter Mac and Melbourne Health, respectively, were the other two large members of the Western and Central Metropolitan Integrated Cancer Services and were both major teaching hospitals of the University of Melbourne. Importantly, they both had very large cancer loads and areas of research excellence.

After extensive and, at times, frustrating discussion, the Ludwig Institute headquarters in New York decided to close its Melbourne branch so Ludwig Institute resigned its membership.

CHAPTER 33

Recently, the Austin Hospital including the Olivia Newton-John Cancer and Wellness Centre and the Murdoch Children's Research Institute have joined the consortium.

Importantly, after an international search, Professor Jim Bishop, at that time the commonwealth Chief Medical Officer, with extensive experience in establishing institutional and state-wide cancer services in New South Wales and extensive clinical and research experience in cancer in Victoria, including at the Peter Mac was appointed as the executive director. His appointment has been critical to the gradual move to the realisation of the aspirations of the centre.

At the time of writing, the building program is well under way and progress is being made towards sorting out the complex governance and finance issues. From baseline census data, it is clear the partners in the joint venture are performing outstandingly well in terms of high citation journal publications, indicating that the research productivity is at the highest international level (in the top ten cancer centres for total contribution to the publications rated in the top 10 per cent in the world on the basis of their impact factor). It is very exciting to contemplate what will be achieved if the partners can work constructively together and form the appropriate relationships with the other major sites of cancer treatment and research in Victoria and Australia.

Another exciting and challenging role is as chair of the Council of EMBL Australia. EMBL and Australia's role as an associate member has been discussed in an earlier chapter.

EMBL Australia is in the process of negotiating its further funding, including a restructure of its relationship with EMBL. It has made great progress and it will be a great pity if the current budget situation in Australia puts its membership renewal at risk.

I am the president of the National Stroke Foundation. This is an impressive not-for-profit organisation which is the peak national body for stroke, dealing with public education, prevention, hospital quality assurance, guidelines for treatment and rehabilitation, advocacy and support for stroke research. Despite it being the second most common cause of death in our community and a leading cause of disability in people of all ages, stroke gets relatively little publicity and very small amounts of specific government program funding. I accepted the invitation to become president of this organisation partly because my father had died of a stroke at the age of thirty-seven and partly because I was so impressed by the passion and ability of its CEO, a speech pathologist, Dr Erin Lalor. She had overseen its growth from a fledgling organisation with about six employees to a most effective national organisation with over seventy employees and a budget of AUS$16 million.

I have enjoyed another interesting role as president of Australian University Sport. This is the umbrella organisation for the sports administration officers in Australia's universities. Under the excellent leadership of Don Knapp and a committed and talented board, it has broadened its activities from its traditional role in staging the Australian University Games and regional lead-up events to additional roles such as campaigning against binge drinking by university students and encouraging sporting and recreational participation on university campuses. It campaigned successfully for the reintroduction of compulsory student amenities and services fees which were essential to strong sporting organisations at universities. At the elite level, it supported the 'elite athlete friendly university' program and did research and published material demonstrating the importance of university athletes to the success of a nation's performance at Olympic Games. It worked closely with the Australian Sports Commission which provided funds for a number of its activities.

I was invited by the chair to join the board of the Florey Neurosciences Institute, a medical research institute which was affiliated with the University of Melbourne and which I knew well as I had had a period on its board when I was dean of the Faculty of Medicine, Dentistry and Health Sciences at the University of Melbourne. New buildings on the University of Melbourne campus and at the Austin Hospital were being completed for the institute and its research partners in neuroscience, including the University of Melbourne, the Mental Health Research Institute, the Austin Hospital and the Royal Melbourne Hospital.

The Mental Health Research Institute was relatively small despite the importance of its work, and with its collocation to the new building housing the Florey Neuroscience Institute, there was a strong argument for amalgamation of the two institutes. This was especially so as the director of the Mental Health Research Institute was Colin Masters, a distinguished researcher in the field of Alzheimer's disease, an area clearly overlapping with work at the Florey. Amalgamations are never easy and there were a number of sensitivities involved in this case. Along with Rob Trenberth from the Florey board, and Rob Gerrand and Andrew Stripp from the board of the Mental Health Research Institute, I was appointed to a negotiating committee chaired

CHAPTER 33

by the dean of the faculty, James Angus. This met at frequent intervals over the next eighteen months and all the issues were gradually resolved. A successful amalgamation occurred to form the Florey Institute of Neuroscience and Mental Health, directed by Geoff Donnan and with a merged board chaired by Harold Mitchell. Rob Trenberth and I stepped down from the board at that time, feeling our work was done.

I also chaired the Research and Education Foundation of the Royal Australasian College of Physicians for three years. During that time, we managed to persuade the council to adopt a voluntary 'opt-out' option to donate to the foundation at the time of the annual subscription, which was highly successful. I felt it appropriate that there should be a separate research committee of the college and that the foundation should be chaired by a board member of the college. I was, therefore, able to step down from this position.

I was invited to come on to the council of my old school, Melbourne Grammar, by the chair, Sandy Clark, in 2007. I was then appointed to succeed him as chair of the council in 2010. It has been a privilege and pleasure as there is an excellent headmaster, Roy Kelley, and the council is highly collegial and competent. Although I am a strong supporter of the public school system, I also think that our system is helped by the diversity and excellence that comes from having a parallel private system. I am pleased to say that the school is broadening access by providing many scholarships (16 per cent of the students are on full or partial scholarships and bursaries), and it runs very successful programs for Indigenous students and students from PNG.

I was invited by Tan Sri Jeffrey Cheah to be a trustee on his education foundation in Malaysia, a role that keeps me in touch with Monash's Malaysian Campus as well as a number of former colleagues from the Monash University Sunway board. The vice-chancellor of the University of South Pacific, Rajesh Chandra, asked me to be an advisor and I visit the university usually once per year as well as meeting Rajesh in Melbourne from time to time. The University is headquartered in Suva and has campuses on many Pacific Islands. I also chair the Victorian selection committee for the Sir John Monash Scholarships.

I was appointed in 2012 as a governor of the Ian Potter Foundation, a wonderful philanthropic trust which distributes over AUS$20 million per year for medical, scientific, education and environmental research and activities, and which supports cultural and community organisations. I am also chairing the holding company for the Australian synchrotron (ASHCo) pending its transfer to the commonwealth.

NEW TRICKS

I have not sought consultancies but have been asked to undertake a number for the commonwealth, for Western Australia and for Monash University and the Universities of Sydney and Adelaide. The minister for community services in Victoria, Mary Wooldridge, asked me to chair an expert advisory group, helping the Victorian government with its new strategy on alcohol and other drugs.

I have recently been appointed to the council of La Trobe University.

I have been very fortunate to have such a varied and interesting portfolio of activities. Monash has generously provided me with an office in its city building, separate from the floors occupied by Monash but supported by Monash ITS and by the city office staff. It provides a wonderful base.

With my range of professional activities, my nine grandchildren, more time for golf and a renewed career as a masters rower after a gap of forty-five years, I am fully occupied and physically and mentally fitter than for many years.

Chapter 34

FINAL REFLECTIONS

I can only reflect on how fortunate I have been to have been born in this country, at this time in history, and to have had the parents, wife and children that I have been blessed with. Add to that, the challenges and stimulation of my career in medicine, teaching, research and health and university administration, and I can think of no more fortunate a life.

Young people often ask me for guidance. I am loathe to be too specific as each person's interests, opportunities and choices will be different. My life was almost completely unplanned. I decided to do medicine late in my school days. I had no intention of being an academic or researcher until three years after graduation and no notion of being a university vice-chancellor until I was almost sixty. Is this the right way to go about things? Not for everyone, but I was fortunate enough that it worked for me.

Clearly, there were three key decision points that had a vast influence on my life and career. The first and most important was the decision I made when young and inexperienced to ask Caroline to marry me and her inexplicable decision to agree despite my earlier disclaimer that I was not going to be one of those doctors who made a lot of money.

My decision to leave my comfortable, well-paid and prestigious position as a consultant at the Royal Melbourne Hospital to join a new university department for considerably less remuneration and prestige at the Repatriation General Hospital in the outer suburbs of Melbourne was a key step that changed my career course. And finally, my late decision to enquire about the position of vice-chancellor at Monash when the appointment process was about to be finalised led to the most challenging and rewarding stage of my professional career.

Some people like to set very specific career goals and to work consistently to achieve them. Such an approach works for many. But opportunities and

NEW TRICKS

obstacles are unpredictable and the alternative philosophy of making clear decisions at the various crossroads that you come upon and pursuing the next venture with passion is a more successful approach for others. In any event, drifting along aimlessly and using financial reward as the sole criterion to drive choice are two avenues to an unfulfilled life.

I feel that I am far from being an old dog, but I am indeed fortunate to have learnt a few tricks along life's intriguing path.

INDEX

Abdul Aziz   41
Aboriginal and Torres Strait Islander Council (ATSIC)   118
Ackland, Tom   14
African National Congress (ANC)   204, 207
Age (newspaper)   61
Alfred Hospital   3
Al-Mahaidi, Dr Riadh   231
American University of Sharjah   233
Amos, Bernard   68–69
Amr   234
Ancora Imparo   170
Anderson, Ian   126
Anderson, John   203, 206
Anderson, Warwick   116–117, 123
Andersson, Arne   29
Andrews, Daniel   105, 249
Angus, James   253
Ariotti, Dallas   117
Arizona State University   223, 227
Asmal, Kader   203
asylum seekers' health   133–134
AusIMed   231
Austin Hospital   105, 251–252
Austin Hospital Department of Medicine   33, 36, 38
Austin Research Institute   11
Australia Israel Chamber of Commerce   229
Australia–China Project   51
Australian Council for Educational Research (ACER)   90–91
Australian Health Care Agreement   62, 123
Australian (newspaper)   116, 145
Australian Health Ministers Advisory Council (AHMAC)   72, 75, 120, 123–124
Australian Learning and Teaching Council   180
Australian Medical Association   69–70
Australian Medical Council (AMC)   69, 71, 75, 78, 82, 200
   Academy of Sport Health and Education   96
   Accreditation Committee (Medical School)   71, 75–80
   Specialist Education Accreditation Committee   76, 79
Australian Medical Workforce Advisory Council (AMWAC)   72
Australian National University (ANU)   236
Australian Regenerative Medicine Institute (ARMI)   174, 213
Australian Research Council (ARC)   162, 171, 173
Australian Sports Commission   252

Australian Synchrotron Holding Company (ASHCo)   254
Australian Technology Network   238
Australian University Sport   252
Australian Vice-Chancellors' Committee (AVCC)   236–240

Baillieu-Napthine government   105
Bangalore   215
Bangladesh   218–219
Bartlett, Helen   192, 201
Batterham, Robin   122
Ben-Gurion University of the Negev   230
Best, Jack   117, 120–121
Bio 21 Cluster   101–103, 139, 196
Bio 21 Institute   103
Bioinformatics Resource Australia EMBL (BRAEMBL)   213
Biopolis   110
Biota   122
Bishop, Jim   251
Blewett, Neal   68
Bond University   3
Botswana   105–106
Bracks-Brumby Labor government   186, 213
Bradley, Denise   242
Bradley Review   237, 242–243
Brewer, Brian   27
Briggs, Paul   96
Brook, Geoff   122
Brown, Gordon   244
Browne, Chris   167, 201
Brumby, John   101, 103, 246
Burnet, Sir Frank Macfarlane   91, 100, 121
Byrne, Ed   166, 193–194, 200, 210–211, 226

Cade, John   10
Cahill, George   26
Cain and Kirner governments   58
Cain, John   104
Campbell, Kate   10
Cape Town   207
Cardiac Society   136
Carr, Kim   213, 240–242, 245
casemix funding   58
Clinical Casemix Advisory Committee   61
Casey, Lord Richard   194
Centre for Drug Candidate Optimisation   197
Centre for Green Chemistry   174
Centre for Jewish Civilisation   187
Ceylon College of Physicians   134–135
Chain, Sir Ernst   122

– 257 –

Chaithiraphan, Supachai   135
Chalmers, Don   117
Chalmers, John   47, 131
Chan, Margaret   144
Chandra, Ramesh   253
Chapman, Bruce   156
Chapman, Colin   197
Charles, Bob   195, 227
Charman, Bill   197
Cheah, Susan   199
Cheah, Tan Sri Jeffrey   198–202, 246, 253
China   51–57, 106, 221–226
Chengdu   221–223
Chinese Academy of Science   224
Chinese Aluminium Company (CHALCO)   221
Chinese University of Hong Kong   144
Chisholm Institute   185
Chulabhorn, HRH Princess   135
Churchill Fellowship   20
Clark, Megan   215
Clark, Sandy   253
Clark, Stella   50, 102
Clarke, Ron   101
Clunie, Gordon   81–82, 86, 93–94
Coaldrake, Peter   245
Coleman, Barbara   27
Coleman, Doug   27
Collins, Vernon   10
Colman, Peter   82
Colombo Plan   198
communication   169–170
continuing medical education (CME) or continuing professional development (CPD)   137–138
Cornish, Edwina   166, 171–173, 212, 215, 246–247
Corryong   2
Cory, Suzanne   100–101, 103
Costello, Peter   243
Costello, Tim   133
cost shifting   62–63
Court, John   37
Crook, Alison   154, 161,164–165, 195
CSIRO   175–176, 186
Cust, Betty   5
Cust, Eric   12
Cutler Review   242, 245

Daines, Doug   1
Dalai Lama   225
Darvall, Peter   141–142, 145, 149, 247
Darwin   69
Davis, David   105
Davis, Glyn   245
Davison, Graeme   210
Dawkins, John   68, 237
Dawkins reforms   185, 237
Delaney, Max   188
De Luca, Hector   25–26
Department of Education, Employment and Workplace Relations (DEEWR)   243
Department of Health (Commonwealth)   69
Department of Health (Victorian)   60
Dias, Reynold   163
Dlamini-Zuma, Nkosazana   208
Doe, William   117
Doherty Committee of Inquiry into Medical Education and the Workforce   68–74, 77
    consumer consultations   69–70
Doherty, Peter   112
Doherty, Ralph   68–70
Donnan, Geoff   253
Doyle, Austin   34, 38–39, 89
Doyle, Jill   38
Duckett, Stephen   62
Duke University   110
Duncan, Jenepher   188
Dunlop, Marjorie   vii, 37, 49–50, 83

Economic Development Board of Singapore   109
Edelsten, Geoffrey   8–9
Education Investment Fund (EIF)   175, 244
education, medical
    continuing medical education (CME) or continuing professional development (CPD)   137–138
    medical education   7–9, 68–71, 77, 82–86
    medical research institutes, affiliation with universities   99
    problem-based learning (PBL)   83–86, 89, 94
    research and scholarship   171–178
    rural clinical schools   73, 96–97, 150
    rural scholarships   74
    selection for medical school   86–88, 90
    teaching-research nexus   180
    unbundling costs of teaching and research in hospitals   124
    university education, quality of   179
    university rankings   179
    see also specific institutions listed by name
Edwards, Kerrie   vii
Elliott, Susan   94, 146
Ellis, Jerry   142–143, 210
EMBL Australia   211–213, 251
Emerson, Craig   240
Endocrine Society of Australia   19, 39, 50
endocrinology   17–19
end of life care   67
Enterprise Agreement (EBA)   168–169
Equiset   154, 189
Eric Susman Prize for Medical Research   39
European Bioinformatics Institute (EBI)   212, 213
European Molecular Biology Laboratory (EMBL)   211–213
Evans, Hugh   183
Evans, Merran   210

INDEX

Ewing, Maurice 9–10
Excellence in Research Australia (ERA) 240

Fahd, Crown Prince 43–44
Fahey, Stephanie 211, 222–223, 227, 247
Faine, John 158
Fairchild, Ron 247
Fairley, Ken 17, 31–32
Family Court 3
Farjou, Nizar 232
Federation University 193, 197
Feeney, Chuck 101
Finkel, Alan 246
Finkel, Ron 231
Fleming, Sir Alexander 122
Flinders Medical Centre 47
Flinders University 86, 131
Flood, Philip 121
Florey Institute of Neuroscience and Mental Health 253
Florey Medal 121
Florey Neuroscience Institute 252
Florey, Sir Howard 121
Fone, David 14, 17
Fraser, Bob 46
Frew, Sir John ('Jock') 14–17, 34, 130
Fudan University 108
Funder, John 114–116

Gandel family 228
Garrett, Geoff 175
General Electric Research Laboratories 215
General Medical Council, UK 76
general physicians 47, 136
Genuth, Saul 27
George, Peter 233
Gerrand, Rob 252
Gilbert, Alan 81, 97, 99, 107, 111, 139–140, 150, 174
Gillard, Julia 66, 240–243
  see also Rudd-Gillard government 66, 238, 241–242
Gilmour, David 206–207
Gippsland Education Precinct 192
Gluckman, Peter 78
Godfrey, Jayne 167
Gonski Review 243
Gosper, Kevan 154–155
Graduate Australian Medical School Admissions Test (GAMSAT) 90
Grollo, Lorenz 154–155, 189
Grollo, Diana 209
Grollo, Rino 154–155, 209
Group of Eight 238
Guilfoyle, Margaret 117

Hadassah Hospital 230–231
Hamilton, John 76
Hammersmith Hospital 20–21, 29
Royal Postgraduate Medical School 20
Harradine, Brian 114
Harris, Peter 94
Hawke-Keating government 156, 237
health care professionals
  general physicians 47–48, 136
  medical workforce 68, 71–74
  nurses 65
health care system, Australia
  casemix funding 58
  Clinical Casemix Advisory Committee 61
  cost shifting 62–63
  crisis in hospitals in Victoria 64–65
  hospital and health care funding 58–67, 124
  Indigenous health
    see National Aboriginal Community Controlled Health Organisations (NACCHO); National Aboriginal and Torres Strait Islander Health Council (NATSIHC)
  length of stay in hospital 63
  mental health services 63–64
  medical negligence 67
  medical workforce 68, 71–74
  throughput bonus pool 60
  unbundling costs of teaching and research in hospitals 124
  see also rural health; hospital; and specific governments, government departments, organisations, programs and initiatives listed by name
Health Research Council, NZ 79
Heaney, Tom 40
Hearn, June 210
Heatley, Norman 121–122
Heidrick and Struggles 142
Hellerstrom, Claes 29
Henderson, Margaret 17
Heyma, Paula 33
Hicks, Neville 68
Higher Education Contribution Scheme (HECS) 153, 156–157, 237, 239
Higher Education Endowment Fund 186, 243
Hill, Rod 177
HIV-AIDS 105, 128, 135
Hone, Sir Brian 4–5
Hong Kong 143–144
hospitals
  casemix funding 58
  Clinical Casemix Advisory Committee 61
  crisis in hospitals in Victoria 64–65
  general physicians 47–48, 136
  hospital and health care funding 58–67, 124
  length of stay in hospital 63
  mental health services 63–64
  medical workforce 68, 71–74

– 259 –

nurses 65
throughput bonus pool 60
unbundling costs of teaching and research in hospitals 124
see also, specific hospitals listed by name
Howard Florey Institute 112
Howard, John 97, 120, 122, 156, 220
   Howard government 73, 238–240, 243, 245
Hudson, Bryan 39, 130
Hunter, Arnold (Puggy) 126–127
Hussain al-Shahristani 231

Ian Potter Foundation 253
Indian Institute of Technology Bombay (IITB) 216–220
IITB-Monash Research Academy 214–220
Indigenous health
   see National Aboriginal Community Controlled Health Organisations (NACCHO); National Aboriginal and Torres Strait Islander Health Council (NATSIHC)
Infosys 215
Innovative Research Universities 238
insulin release 19
International Congress of Endocrinology 39
International Olympic Committee (IOC) 154–155
Israel 229

Jackson, Daryl 101
Jewish Civilisation, Centre for 228
Jinan 51, 55, 57
Jiuzhaigou National Park 223
Joan Rosanove Chambers 2
Johnston, Colin 61
Johnston, Ian 177
Joseph, Sarah 225
Joslin Clinic 27
Juttoddie 6–7

Kadir, Khalid 201
Karpin, David 104
Kelley, Roy 253
Kemp, Celia 117
Kemp, David 117
Kempler, Leon 229
Kent, Bill 209
Kennett, Jeff 59, 64–65, 133
   Kennett government 64
Kincaid-Smith, Priscilla 10–11, 32–33, 45, 46, 89
King, Max 222
King's College London 210
Knapp, Don 252
Kosky, Lynne 195
Kovacs, Gab 177
KPMG 124
Krishnamoorthy, Mohan 220
Krongold family 228

Lacy, Paul 27
Lalor, Erin 252
Lancet (journal) 25, 28
Larkins, Bill 1
Larkins, Chlothilde 1
Larkins, Caroline viii, 11–12, 15–16, 21–24, 28,32, 34–35, 55–56, 81, 135, 249, 255
Larkins, Fiona vii, 21
Larkins, Frank 99–100
Larkins, Graeme 1–3
Larkins, John 1, 20
Larkins, Kate viii, 28
Larkins, Richard
   China 1985 51–57
   Doherty Committee 68–73
   early years and background 1–5
   education 3–4, 6–13
   EMBL Australia 213
   engagement and wedding 11–12
   Monash University
      appointment to 139–147
      early days 148–155
      farewell to 247–249
      life after 250–255
      student riots 156–160
   Medical Schools Accreditation Committee, AMC 74–80
   National Aboriginal and Torres Strait Islander Health Council (NATSIHC) 125–128
   National Health and Medical Research Council, Chair 114–124
   PhD thesis 27–28
   Royal Australasian College of Physicians, presidency of 129–138
   Royal Postgraduate Medical School, PhD student at 21–30
   private medical practice 33, 146–147
   Repatriation General Hospital, Heidelberg 36–40
   Royal Melbourne Hospital
      assistant endocrinologist 17–20
      clinical training 14–20
      James Stewart Chair of Medicine 45–50
      physician to the endocrine laboratory 31
      physician to outpatients 31
      senior medical staff, member of 31–40
   Saudi Arabia 41–44
   Sir Arthur Simms Commonwealth Travelling Professorship 81, 83
   Universities Australia, Chair 237–246
   University of Melbourne
      Dean, Faculty of Medicine, Dentistry and Health Sciences 93–113
      Deputy Dean 81–92
   University of Sharjah, Board of

INDEX

Trustees 234–235
Larkins, Sarah vii, 22, 28
Larkins, Stephen 1
Larson, Gary vii, 37
La Trobe University 254
Lazarus, Mark 2
Learning and Teaching Performance Fund 179
Lee, Weng Keng 201
Leeder, Stephen 116–117
Leeton, John 177
Liberman, Lee 228, 230
Liddell, Merilyn 200–201
Lindenderry 98
Lindsay, Alan 167
Little, Peter 41
Logan, Mal 196, 235
Lomax-Smith Review 237, 243
long-acting thyroid stimulator (LATS, TSI) 18
Lopata, Alex 177
Lovell, Richard 9, 18–19, 33–34, 45, 47, 89
Lucas, Arthur 210
Ludwig Institute 249–250
Lusink, Peg viii, 1–3
Lusink, Theo 3

Maastricht University 85
MacCauley, Seamus 25
MacIntyre, Mabs 22, 38–39
MacIntyre, Iain 20, 22, 25–26, 29, 37–38
Mackay, Ian 48
Macklin, Jenny 63
Macleish, Scotty 14
Magdalen College Oxford 121
Maisela, Max 204, 208
Marshall, Peter 148, 168, 189, 220, 247
Martin, Christine 34
Martin, Ian ('Skip') 17–19, 82
Martin, Jack 33–34, 37, 39, 45, 61
Mashelkar, Ramesh 218
Masters, Colin 252
Matheson, Sir Louis 159
Mattaj, Iain 212–213
Mayo Clinic 26
McCarthy, John 218, 220
McCaughey, Patrick 188
McGauran, Peter 193
McGill University 83
McKenzie, Brian 190, 192
McKenzie, Ian CF 11, 27
McKenzie, Ian H 11
McMaster University 83
McPhee, Peter 8
Medical Workforce Data Review Committee 72
Medicare 66, 68, 73–74
medicine, areas of research and treatment
   endocrinology 17–19
   end of life care 67
   insulin release 19
   long-acting thyroid stimulator (LATS, TSI) 18
   mental health services 63–64
   pancreatic islet transplantation 27, 29–30, 53–54
   prolactin 19
   traditional Chinese medicine 54–56
   vitamin D metabolism 23, 29, 39
Melbourne Centre for Nanofabrication 178
Melbourne Grammar School 1, 4, 252
Melbourne Health 250
   see Royal Melbourne Hospital
Melick, Roger 46
Mental Health Research Institute 252
mental health services 63–64
Menzies Centre 210
Menzies government 236
Michelangeli, Valdo 40
Miller, Loren 220
Misra, Ashok 216, 220
Mitchell, Harold 253
Mobilio, Liz vii, 146
Monash University 4, 11, 39, 87, 106, 140–141, 146, 148–235, 255
   academic board 166–167
   Accident Research Centre 174, 246
   administration and finance 161–170
   Senior Management Committee (SMC) 166
   strategic cost management (SCM) 161–163
   Architecture, School of 187
   Berwick campus 149, 185, 194
   Caulfield campus 149, 185, 187–190
   China 222–227
   Clayton campus 149, 185–186
   Committee of Deans 166
   David Derham School of Law 189
   David Syme Business School 185
   Gippsland campus 149–150, 164, 185, 190–193
      Gippsland medical school 192–193
   India 214–221
   Institute for Global Movements 174
   Institute for Pharmaceutical Sciences 174
   Jeffrey Cheah School of Medicine 201
   London Centre 154, 210–211
   Malaysia (Sunway campus) 106, 246
   matrix management 191
   Melbourne-Monash protocol 174
   Monash College 164
   Monash IVF 177
   Monash Passport 183
   Monash Property Management (MPM) 164
   Monash University Museum of Art

(MUMA)   187–188
MonCom   164, 176
Monyx   165
Occupational Therapy, School of   194
Peninsula campus   149, 185, 193–194
Pharmacy College (Parkville)   196–197
Physiotherapy, School of   194
Prato Centre   154, 209–210
shootings   142
specialist science high school   186
statement of purpose   153
student riots at Monash   156–160
South Africa   141, 164, 203–208, 246
Student Association (MSA)   150, 157–160
Sustainability Institute   174
Vice-Chancellor's Group (VCG)   151, 166, 168
Morey, Sue   68
Morstyn, George   250
Mothlante, Kgalema   207
Mount Royal Hospital   3
Muddle, Barry   224
Muirden, Ken   45
Mullarvey, John   240
Mumbai   216
terrorist attacks   220
Murdoch Children's Research Institute   105, 251
Murray Committee   236–237
Murray, Sir Keith   236
Murray, Shane   187
Murthy, Naryana   215

Nanyang Technical University   110
National Aboriginal Community Controlled Health Organisations (NACCHO)   126
National Aboriginal and Torres Strait Islander Health Council (NATSIHC)   122, 125–128
National Cancer Institute   250
National Collaborative Research Infrastructure Strategy   242
National Health and Medical Research Council (NHMRC)   29, 50, 111, 114–124, 127, 131, 162, 171, 173
 Australian Health Ethics Committee   114, 116
 Health Advisory Committee   114, 116
 Research Committee   114, 116
 Strategic Research Advisory Committee (SRAC)   117
National Press Club   245
National Registration and Training Scheme   75
National Stroke Foundation   251
National University Hospital Singapore   110
National University of Singapore   108
Nature (journals)   19, 28
Neher, Erwin   111–112

Nelson, Brendan   156
'reforms'   156, 241
Newman, Louise   134
New Zealand Medical Council   78–79
New Zealand Obese (NZO) mice   18–19, 39
Niall, Hugh   27, 40,122
Noad, Sir Kenneth   130
Nobel Prize   111–113
Nolan, Terry   96
Nouri al-Maliki   232
Norris, Rob   215, 219
Nossal High School   195
Nossal, Sir Gustav   46, 100, 195
nurses   65

Oaktree Foundation   183
O'Dea, Kerin   49–50
Olivia Newton-John Cancer and Wellness Centre   251
Orr, Sidney   8
Oxburgh, Lord Ron   109
Oz-Salzberger, Fania   228

Palmer, Gill   208
pancreatic islet transplantation   27, 29–30, 53–54
Papua New Guinea   130
Parhar, Ishwar   201
Parker, Stephen   145, 148–149, 152, 158–159, 165–166, 168, 177,183, 209, 247
Parkville precinct (strip)   103, 196
Patterson, Craig   132, 134
Peking University Health Science Centre   106
Penington, David   50, 61, 66, 76, 81–82, 102, 104, 133, 196
Peter MacCallum Cancer Clinic (Centre)   9, 103–105, 249–250
Phang, Koon Tuck   201
Pharmaceutical Benefits Scheme   62
Phillips, David   153
Piterman, Leon   196, 232
Pitt, David   164, 177, 189, 247
Podger, Andrew   125
policy *see* health care system, Australia
Pollard, Robin   201
Pollock, Andrew   159
Potts, John   40
Pratt family   228
Pretorius, Tyrone   206–207
Prime Minister's Science, Engineering and Innovation Council (PMSEIC)   122–123, 244
Prince Henry's Hospital   11
Princess Marina Hospital, Gaborone   105
problem-based learning (PBL)   83–86, 89, 94
Proietto, Joe   49
prolactin   19
provost, role of   139, 165

INDEX

Pumphrey, David 142
Purdue University 227

Queensland University of Technology 245

Ramler, Paul 204
Rank, Sir Benjamin 9–10
Rao, C.N.R. 216–217
Razak, Najib 201
Redman, John 187
Renold, Albert 24
Repatriation General Hospital
   Heidelberg 33–40, 255
research
   medical research institutes 99
   research assessment exercise
     (RAE) 242
   research and scholarship 171–178
   teaching-research nexus 180
   unbundling costs of teaching and research
     in hospitals 124
   see also specific research bodies and
     programs listed by name
Reynolds, Eric 97
Roberts, Ken 131
Robinson, David 141, 143, 152, 154, 164, 166, 174, 203, 210, 247
Rogers, Susie 40
Rogge, Jacques 155
Rosenberg, John 154
Rosanove, Edward 1
Rosanove, Joan 1
Rosenberg, John 154
Rosenthal, Nadia 211–213
Rossjohn, Jamie 172
Roth, Jesse 27
Royal Australasian College of Physicians
   (RACP) 17, 32, 37, 39, 41, 50, 115, 129–138, 253
   Health Policy Unit 132
   illicit drug policy 132
   Maintenance of Professional Standards
     (MOPS) 138
   Research and Education
     Foundation 131, 253
Royal Children's Hospital 105, 250
Royal College of Physicians of
   Thailand 134–135
Royal Melbourne Hospital 14–20, 31–35, 57, 64, 100–101, 103–105, 146, 249–250, 252, 255
Royal Women's Hospital 105
RU 486 114
Rudd, Kevin 66, 123, 202, 240–242, 244–245
   see also Rudd-Gillard
     government 66, 238, 241–242
Rumbalara Football and Netball Club 96
Rumsfeld, Donald 84
rural health

rural clinical schools—73, 96–97, 150
rural health departments—73, 96
rural scholarships—74

Ryan, Graeme 50, 81–82, 93–94, 196

Saddam, Hussein 231–232
Sakmann, Bert 111–113
Sakmann, Christianne 112
Sargent, Delys 68
SARS 144
Saudi Arabia 41–44
Saunders, Nick 138, 142–143, 194
Schedvin, Boris 100
scholarship *see* education; research
Schumacher, Silke 212–213
Shandong Province 51–52
Shanghai Jiaotong University 111, 221
Sharjah 232–233
Sharma, M.M. 217
Sheikh Mohammed 232, 234
Sheil, M. 240
Shen 150–151, 158–160
Shepparton 96–97
Shi, Jian 223
Shoemaker, Adam 183, 247
Sibal, Kapil 218
Sichuan University 221–223
Simmons, David 96
Simms Commonwealth Travelling
   Professor 81, 83
Singapore 109–110
Singapore General Hospital 110
Smallwood, Richard (Dick) 76, 89, 114–115
Smith, Robert 69
Smith, Tony 121
Spittle, Stanley 101
Sri Lanka 135
Sridhar, Tam 215, 220
Stanley, Fiona 244–245
St David's School 3
Steele, Philip 196
St Jude's Hospital 113
St Vincent's Hospital 105, 250
Stewart, David 79
Stewart, Doff 79
Stockdale, Alan 59
Stojanovska, Lily 40
Stripp, Andrew 252
Sultan bin Mohammed Al-Qasimi 232–234
Sunway Group 199
Sutton, Gerard 239–240
Swan, Wayne 242
Synchrotron 149, 172, 178, 186

Tai Shan 56
Tan Chorh Chan 109
Tan, Tony 109
Tanner, Lindsay 240

teaching-research nexus   180
Tehan, Marie   61
Tertiary Education Quality and Standards Authority (TEQSA)   243
Thomson Learning   108–109
Thrift, Nigel   211
throughput bonus pool   60
Townsend, Sir Lance   10
Townsville   69
traditional Chinese medicine   54–56
training *see* education
Trainor, Rick   210
Tregear, Geoff   27, 40
Trenberth, Rob   252–253
Trounson, Alan   177

U 21   108–109
U 21 Global   108–109, 139
Undergraduate Medical and Health Professions Admission Test (UMAT)   91–92
Universities Australia   236–245
University of Auckland   78, 108
University of Ballarat   193, 197
University of Birmingham   108, 117
University of Botswana   105, 206
University of British Columbia   83, 108
University of Calcutta   219
University of Calgary   83, 84
University of Cambridge   172
University of Canberra   149
University of Cardiff   172
University of Dhaka   218
University of Edinburgh   108
University of Glasgow   108
University of Hong Kong   108
University of Leiden   154
University of Manchester   140
University of Melbourne   4, 6–13, 81–92, 104–105, 146, 149–150, 163, 174–175, 181, 249, 252
    advanced medical sciences   95
    dental school   82, 97
    James Stewart Chair of Medicine   45
    Janet Clarke Hall   6, 11–12
    Nursing, School of Postgraduate   82
    Melbourne Business School   107
    Melbourne model   181
    Melbourne-Monash protocol   174
    Melbourne University Private   107, 109, 139
    Physiotherapy, School of   82
    Population Health, School of   95
    Trinity College   6–7, 11, 112
University of Newcastle   76, 83, 85
University of New South Wales   108
University of Nottingham   108
University of Otago   78–79
University of Ottawa   83
University of Pune   219
University of Queensland   76, 86, 108
University of Sharjah   233
University of Southern Queensland   190
University of South Pacific   253
University of Sydney   86
University of Toronto   83
University of Western Cape   207
University of Wollongong   239–240
university rankings   179
Undergraduate Research Opportunities Program (UROP)   103

Vanstone, Amanda   156, 239
    'cuts'   156–157, 239
Victorian Comprehensive Cancer Centre   105, 249
Viravaidya, Mechai   135
vitamin D metabolism   23, 29, 39

Walker, Sally   108, 139–140, 193
Wallace, David   111
Walter and Eliza Hall Institute   18, 46, 48, 100–101, 104
Wang de Quan   57
Wark, John   40
Warwick University   211
Watters, Brian   133
Webb, Graham   152, 180
Webb, John   218
Welch, Jack   215
Wellington, Heather   104
Western and Central Metropolitan Integrated Cancer Services (WCMICS)   250
Western Hospital   105, 250
Whelan, Greg   89
Whitlam government   237
Whitworth, Judith   123
Whisstock, James   172
Wilcock, Ian   204, 208
Williams, Roland   102
Wills, Peter   120
Wills Review   120, 122, 239
Wilson Transformer Company   176
Withers, Glenn   240, 242
Wodak, Alex   133
Wood, Carl   177
Wooldridge, Mary   254
Wooldridge, Michael   73, 96, 114–117, 120, 125
World Health Organisation (WHO)   144
Wright, Sir Roy Douglas ('Pansy')   8, 46

Xie, Heping   222–223

Yeo, Philip   109

Zaini, Anuar   200–201
Zimbabwe   208
Zinkernagel, Rolf   113
Zinn, Shirley   204
Zuma, Jacob   208